The
Exhaustion
Cure

Also by Laura Stack

Find More Time: How to Get Things Done at Home, Organize Your Life, and Feel Great About It

Leave the Office Earlier: The Productivity Pro Shows You How to Do More in Less Time . . . and Feel Great About It

The Exhaustion Cure

UP Your Energy
from LOW to GO in 21 Days

Laura Stack

BROADWAY BOOKS
NEW YORK

PUBLISHED BY BROADWAY BOOKS

Published in the United States by Broadway Books, an imprint of The Doubleday
Broadway Publishing Group, a division of Random House, Inc., New York.
www.broadwaybooks.com

BROADWAY BOOKS and its logo, a letter B bisected on the diagonal, are trademarks of
Random House, Inc.

Book design by Diane Hobbing of Snap-Haus Graphics

Library of Congress Cataloging-in-Publication Data
Stack, Laura.
   The Exhaustion cure : up your energy from low to go in 21 days / Laura Stack. —
1st ed.
      p. cm.
   1. Vitality. 2. Fatigue—Prevention. 3. Health. 4. Mental health. 5. Self-care,
Health. I. Title.

RA776.95.S69 2008
613—dc22
2007030179

ISBN 978-0-7679-2751-2

PRINTED IN THE UNITED STATES OF AMERICA

10 9 8 7 6 5 4 3 2

To my Baby Girl,
Meagan Stack,
whose love,
beautiful heart, and spirit
always give me energy

Contents

PART 1 • PHYSIOLOGY • 21

ONE • Sleep • 23

TWO • Diet • 38

THREE • Nutrition • 58

FOUR • Exercise • 81

PART 2 • PRACTICES • 131

EIGHT • Quick Fixes • 133

ENERGY BANDITS

NINE • Relaxation • 147

ENERGY BANDITS

PART 3 • PERIPHERY • 227

FIFTEEN • Environment • 229

ENERGY BANDITS

SIXTEEN • Relationships • 243

ENERGY BANDITS

SEVENTEEN • Stress • 258

ENERGY BANDITS

EIGHTEEN • Technology • 273

ENERGY BANDITS

NINETEEN · Purpose · 287

TWENTY · Workplace · 300

TWENTY-ONE • Clutter • 315

A Note to Readers

This book is not intended to replace the advice and treatment of a physician. The information, data, behavioral recommendations, tools, and materials in this book are provided for your education and reference only and are not, nor are they intended to be, a medical or psychological evaluation, examination, advice, consultation, diagnosis, or treatment. Any use of the information set forth herein is entirely at the reader's discretion. The author and publisher advise that a person using this manual consult a physician and/or healthcare provider for all medical and health-related matters and have the medical tests necessary to rule out or identify serious disease. If you are presently undergoing treatment for some condition and want to use this manual to augment those methods, please discuss this with your doctor or licensed health professional.

Because every person's health is different, there is always some risk involved in self-treatment. Please do not use this book if you are unwilling to assume that risk. The author and publisher are not responsible for any adverse effects or consequences resulting from the use of any information, products, preparations, or procedures described in this book. The author and the publisher will not be liable for, and you waive any claim for, any personal injury, damage, and/or liability arising out of your reading and your use of or reliance on this book.

Acknowledgments

Since this is my third published book, I can't help feeling a bit redundant in my acknowledgments. But I truly would not be able to be a mom, wife, business owner, speaker, and author without the support of a lot of people. Many people ask me how I can "do it all." I don't. My hero and husband, John, is my rock and the family anchor that keeps things stable when my life is crazy. I am lucky to have a partner who "gets" it.

My children—Meagan, twelve; Johnny, eight; and James, six—are years older now than when I penned my first book, and they are starting to understand what I'm doing when I disappear for days at a time. My love goes out to them for their support while "Mommy is on one of her crazy writing retreats." Even though they miss me, they know writing gives me joy and let me leave without too much hassle. I hope they always remember visiting at my hotel while I'm on retreat, jumping on my bed, and swimming in the pool.

There are a few people in my life I couldn't function without. One is my mother-in-law, Eileen Stack, who selflessly gives her time to help our family. You should count yourself lucky if you have someone in your life like Eileen, who loves you, is devoted to your success, and works tirelessly to help you. Another is my mentor, Dianna Booher, CSP, CPAE, who has coached me month after month for years now and helped me avoid many stumbling blocks. Dianna has written more than 40 books (www.booherdirect.com)—so I have a long way to go to catch up to her—but she encourages me to keep writing. My personal assistant, Dana Hill, is so patient and flexible and handles a million little details for me. Our best friends, Darla and Mark Sanborn (www.marksanborn.com), keep us rooted with their encouragement, laughter, and play time. Thank you for your love and support.

Thanks to my editor from Broadway Books, Becky Cole, for your support and enthusiasm for this book idea. I appreciate the wise counsel of my literary agent, Robert Shepard. When I first met Robert, I was so impressed by his immediate response and organization. He continues to be the perfect agent and a great friend.

Last, most of all, my eternal gratitude goes to my Lord, Jesus Christ, for continuing to shower His blessings upon my life.

The
Exhaustion
Cure

Does the mere thought of embarking on a program to get more energy leave you totally exhausted? Then you might want to read this lying down. "I would love to be more productive!" a reader of one of my first books lamented. "But I'm so exhausted at the end of the day, it's all I can do to get dinner on the table, put the kids to bed, and crash in front of the television. I have no desire to work on projects around the house, much less exercise or think about organizing the garage."

It's a common complaint. Lack of energy is a major culprit at work as well: people sleepwalk through the day, fuzzy-headed and lethargic. Nothing sounds more attractive than putting your head down on your desk for a quick nap. How can you possibly begin that big project that requires high levels of creativity and concentration? Yuck. You'd rather stick pins in your eyes.

You might know all the productivity tips in the world, but nothing will work if you don't have the energy to give 100 percent. Personal energy is a measure of how strong, invigorated, or up to a task you may feel at any moment. Nobody has an unlimited supply of personal energy. If you feel down, your zest ebbs and you'll produce mediocre work. In periods of low energy, your productivity sinks, because you feel like you're slogging through a field of waist-high mud.

My audiences and readers of my two other books, *Find More Time* and *Leave the Office Earlier,* asked me to write this book. "What are you on?" they teased. "Where in the world do you get that much energy?" I didn't realize my trademark energy was such a key component of my productivity level. But the more I observed the habits and energy levels of productive people, the more I understood how vital your vigor is to your performance. You simply cannot perform if you have no drive or desire—the oomph—to be productive. You may find yourself daydreaming about your goals and all the wonderful things you could do if you could just get up and go; but daydreaming and actually having the energy to *do* things are completely different.

I'm going to show you how to get the energy you need to live a full and productive life. You don't have to suffer from low energy. I don't purport to cure any medical conditions, but with consistent applications of the tips outlined in this book, you will realize a huge boost in your energy level—whatever that is for you.

Different people have different energy levels. Some people have the energy to work all day and then run around and clean the house in the evening. Others drag themselves onto the sofa and watch television all night. While it's true that some people have higher natural energy levels, those with lower energy can use personal energy-management techniques to make up the difference. The good news is that you really can change your energy level.

This book is different from other energy books because it takes a holistic, comprehensive approach to energy, not simply a diet approach, or a stress approach, or a spiritual approach. It helps you look at all the "boosters" you need to become energetic—and beat all the "bandits" that conspire to rob you of your energy every day.

Energy Defined

The word *energy* is kicked around quite a bit and has many loose usages, so let's make sure we're on the same page. Let's start by specifying what I *don't* mean by energy.

ENERGY IS NOT TIME. Energy is often equated with time, as in "This project will require a great deal of time and energy." You may have the time, but lacking the energy, the project won't succeed.

You could have all the time in the world but still not feel like doing much.

ENERGY IS NOT HEALTH. For some people, feeling better might lead to more motivation. But plenty of healthy people still have incredibly low energy, thanks to factors that are sapping their strength. For example, if you don't get a good night's sleep, you won't have the energy you need. And while most of us know that a calorie is defined as "a unit of energy-producing potential," some foods can actually decrease your energy level rather than raise it. If you're perfectly healthy but don't eat right or get enough sleep, your energy levels will suffer.

ENERGY IS NOT EMOTION. These two words are also commonly paired, as in "She delivered the speech with energy and emotion." Which part was the energy and which was the emotion? You can definitely have one without the other. Some very energetic people don't show much emotion. And some very emotional people don't have the energy to get off the couch. They *feel* things to an extreme but don't accomplish as much as they'd like to.

ENERGY IS NOT MOTIVATION. Some very energetic people don't feel motivated to work very hard. Indeed, they may be motivated to sit in front of their computers playing solitaire all day.

ENERGY IS NOT PRODUCTIVITY. Are you surprised to hear me say that? You could have all the energy in the world and still not be productive, due to procrastination, lack of skills, unavailable resources, and so forth. (My other books, *Leave the Office Earlier* and *Find More Time,* address how to be productive.) With that said, energy is most closely tied to productivity, because one doesn't easily coexist without the other. If you have energy, you at least have the *ability* to be productive.

So . . . what *is* energy?

ENERGY IS CAPACITY. Physics teaches us that energy is the capacity of a physical system to do work—to carry on the activities that it was designed to accomplish. The human body is a physical system, and we all must work, whether in an office or at home. Every physical system possesses a certain amount of energy; its presence—or absence—allows us to predict how much work the system has the capacity to do. Your capacity to work is your potential ability to work or perform. So for the purposes of this book:

Energy gives you the ability to work. Your **energy level** measures your capacity to put forth productive effort. As your energy levels increase, so will your potential to accomplish your short- and long-term goals and activities.

This capacity could be very high or very low—and of course having the capacity doesn't necessarily mean you will *do* anything. But if you have energy, you at least possess the raw materials necessary to accomplish what you want or need to accomplish; or, as Rudyard Kipling put it, "Enough work to do, and strength enough to do the work." It's when your energy is highest that you're most aroused and capable of sustaining your activity. Think of yourself as a factory. Do you have the energy to operate at 100 percent of capacity? Only 80 percent? What if you were able to acquire more raw materials? Would your "factory" be able to produce more?

Your capacity, energy, and productivity aren't cast in stone; they can and do change. In fact, your capacity to be productive rises and falls throughout the day, and often by the hour or even by the minute, depending upon changes in your energy level. The presence or absence of energy will definitely have an impact on what you're capable of achieving. That's why this book will often talk about energy and productivity together. But it's important to remember that they're two separate things—energy is the source of productivity. As you increase your energy level, you'll be able to accomplish more at work or at home.

Your Sources of Energy

When you begin to explore the causes of your lack of energy, it may be helpful to think of a bank account. Some of our activities or actions are like deposits that give us more energy; but others are like withdrawals that drain our energy. I call the deposits "Energy Boosters" and the drains "Energy Bandits." You would like more deposits in your bank account than withdrawals; in fact, you'd like your balance to be as high as possible.

What gives you energy and what saps your energy? Let's start by brainstorming a master list, in no particular order, and with no particular focus. I'll provide some examples from my own life:

▲Energy Deposits | BOOSTERS

Kisses from my children

A long, hot bath at the end of the day

Sunshine

Walking my dog

Yoga

Talking with my best friend

Sudoku puzzles

Peppermint tea

Spas! Visiting any spa!

Massage

▼Energy Drains | BANDITS

Arguing with my children

No "me" activities

Cloudy, dreary weather

Working late into the evening

No food in the refrigerator

Being overwhelmed or disorganized

My dog has an accident on the floor

A dirty house

Feeling lonely

Too much travel

Not spending enough time with my husband

It's time for you to brainstorm your boosters and bandits. At this point, don't worry about assigning values to these factors. Simply let your mind explore every aspect of your life, from the everyday to the exceptional. What gives you energy and what saps your energy? Feel free to continue this list on a piece of paper or create a master document in a word processing or spreadsheet program.

▲Energy Deposits | BOOSTERS

▾**Energy Drains | BANDITS**

Energy In/Energy Out

Since you haven't weighted these factors and are often comparing minor to major things, this list can't really tell you whether your bank account has a balance—or is overdrawn. But it can get you thinking about the values you'll assign to these factors later on. Remember: your ultimate goal is to have more deposits than drains overall. Do you feel like you have more energy coming in or going out in your life? Since you purchased this book, I'm guessing that your energy account is depleted—and you're in the red.

How is this affecting your productivity? Have you had the capacity to get things done lately? Is your performance suffering? Are you working to your highest ability? Consider how it would look if you were fully energized and your energy account were full. Would it take you less time to complete tasks? Would you accomplish more? Would you feel like starting new projects? Once your energy account is in the black, you will have a higher capacity to be productive.

Organization of the Book

Many of the energy books I've read make it too complicated for a person to learn how to boost their energy levels by distinguishing the type of energy: physical, mental, intellectual, spiritual, and so on. I don't separate energy in this sense, since they're all so closely related. For example, if I'm sleepy (physical), I won't be able to concentrate (intellectual), and I probably shouldn't be getting into heated conversations with my spouse (emotional). If you've ever dragged home exhausted from a marathon workday, only to be instantly revived by your pet's wagging tail, a hug from your child, or a kiss from your spouse, you know being energized goes far beyond what you had for lunch. Instead, I take a broader approach to energy and focus on the *source* of low energy in three main parts:

1. **Physiology:** How your *body* affects your energy—the impact of your health, nutrition, and self-care on how well you feel.

2. **Practices:** How your *behavior* affects your energy—your daily habits surrounding your schedule, choices, and actions.

3. **Periphery:** How your *background* affects your energy—the impact of your environment and external factors, both in and out of your control.

Each section has seven chapters, for a total of twenty-one chapters, each describing one energy factor. Each factor has eight bandits and boosters. Your mission (should you choose to accept it) is to minimize the bandits and maximize the boosters for each factor. For every bandit, I've given you more than one booster to consider.

The Quiz

You'll start by taking the Energy Quotient (EQ) Assessment immediately following this introduction, which outlines the twenty-one energy factors you'll be addressing. You'll rate the extent to which each factor exists in your life. If a factor plays a major role in your life, it's probably an energy booster, and you'll score higher. If the factor is absent, however, its absence becomes an actual drain on your energy—a bandit—which will lower your score. You'll assess all twenty-one factors on a scale of one to five, resulting in a cumulative score based on 105 points. A higher score means a higher energy level. You will quickly see which factors are bandits, robbing you of your energy, and which are boosters. Then your task will be clear: to emphasize energy boosters and, wherever possible, to turn bandits into boosters.

The Program

You can approach the book in one of three ways:

1. **Take a "read what you need" approach.** Use the quiz to identify areas where you need an energy boost and simply turn straight to those sections for concrete suggestions and myriad ways to up your energy in the areas it's being drained.

2. **Take a weekly approach.** Each week, focus on one of the three main areas of energy drain: physiology, practices, and periphery. You'll commit to reading a section of the book over the period of a week. You'll make a variety of changes that work for you and commit to working on them until they become habits. Challenge yourself to raise your EQ by a particular number of points, for example 10 to 50 percent. You can mix and match tips from all of the chapters in that area to get to the right number of points that week. For example, let's say you rated yourself pretty high in the physiology chapters, but your nutrition and sleep scores were low. It would be your job to pick out the boosters that will help you get your physiology score up to your goal by working on nutrition and sleep boosters for as long as you need to make the tips that worked become habits. You don't even have to read for three weeks straight. Start a week-long program as soon as you feel you have the ideas from the previous section under control.

3. **Take a daily approach.** This approach is the most involved. You'll read one chapter each day for twenty-one days in a row, focusing on a single energy factor. That's it. One per day. Each day, you'll read the next chapter, which gives a detailed description of a new energy factor and possible tools for change. You will incorporate one new energy behavior or take

one action each day, either reducing a bandit in your life or adding a booster. This single step will increase the balance in your Energy Account. You may make minimal changes on days where you've already incorporated the advice into your life. Some days, however, will require you to reflect on how you might make a more dramatic change in your habits.

You might even want to create a daily chart, writing out your thoughts on your bandits, boosters, goals, and an action step to help you remember your strategy. A sample chart follows, to give you an idea of what a completed one could look like.

▼ BANDITS. My energy drains in this area:

▲ BOOSTERS. My energy deposits in this area:

My energy goal in this area
(reduce the bandit or increase the booster):

My energy action step for today:

Whatever method you choose, you will become more energetic through changes that individually seem simple but cumulatively make a big difference. By using the boosters in this book, you'll overhaul your energy in a way that fits your lifestyle and preferences, a surefire formula to be at your productive best. Stick with it and, over time, this really *could* cure your energy problems. No time of year is better than another. The ideal time to start is right now.

The Energy Quotient
(EQ) Assessment

Read each of the 21 statements that follow. Circle the number that most closely corresponds to the extent to which you agree with the statement (5 is high; 1 is low). Subtotal your answers for each of the three parts (items 1 through 7: physiology; items 8 to 14: practices; and items 15 through 21: periphery). Total the subtotals from each part to arrive at your grand total, which is your Energy Quotient (EQ).

ENERGY QUIZ | PHYSIOLOGY

	to no extent	to a little extent	to some extent	to a considerable extent	to a great extent
1. I get plenty of sleep at night.	1	2	3	4	5
2. I eat balanced meals and maintain a healthy diet.	1	2	3	4	5
3. I avoid using caffeine or stimulants; I get all the right nutrients my body needs.	1	2	3	4	5

	to no extent	to a little extent	to some extent	to a considerable extent	to a great extent
4. I get sufficient exercise and have strong muscles.	1	2	3	4	5
5. I have a high metabolism.	1	2	3	4	5
6. I experience consistent levels of energy throughout the day.	1	2	3	4	5
7. I take good care of my health and get regular checkups.	1	2	3	4	5

Subtotal Physiology _____

ENERGY QUIZ | PRACTICES

	to no extent	to a little extent	to some extent	to a considerable extent	to a great extent
8. When my energy is low, I know exactly what to do to get going again.	1	2	3	4	5
9. I rest, relax, and pamper myself on a regular basis.	1	2	3	4	5
10. I maintain a great attitude; I think positively rather than negatively.	1	2	3	4	5

	to no extent	to a little extent	to some extent	to a considerable extent	to a great extent
11. I eliminate things in my life that irritate me; I don't tolerate much.	1	2	3	4	5
12. I communicate openly with others to avoid misunderstandings and wasted time.	1	2	3	4	5
13. I consistently accomplish high-value tasks.	1	2	3	4	5
14. I feel challenged every day and I learn continuously.	1	2	3	4	5

Subtotal Practices _____

ENERGY QUIZ | PERIPHERY

	to no extent	to a little extent	to some extent	to a considerable extent	to a great extent
15. I feel energized by my environment, such as lighting, temperature, noise, smell, and furniture.	1	2	3	4	5
16. I have people and relationships in my life that lift me up.	1	2	3	4	5

	to no extent	to a little extent	to some extent	to a considerable extent	to a great extent
17. I feel like I'm in control of my life.	1	2	3	4	(5)
18. I turn off technology regularly; I spend much of my free time involved in nontechnological activities.	1	2	3	(4)	5
19. I follow my purpose or mission in life.	1	2	3	4	5
20. I avoid letting workplace annoyances, such as meetings and interruptions, dictate my schedule.	1	(2)	3	4	5
21. Keep the clutter in my life at bay; I have organized surroundings.	1	2	3	4	5

Subtotal Periphery _25_

TOTAL YOUR SCORES

Subtotal Physiology _21_
+ Subtotal Practices _23_
+ Subtotal Periphery _25_

= GRAND TOTAL _69_

YOUR ENERGY ACCOUNT BALANCE _____

SCORING

89-105	ENDLESS ENERGY! You should be helping others!
72-88	Minor improvements are necessary. Add more Energy Boosters.
55-71	AVERAGE ENERGY. Kick it up a notch.
38-54	Major improvements required. Bust those Energy Bandits!
21-37	RED FLAG! You're being robbed by Energy Bandits!

Part One
PHYSIOLOGY

One

Sleep

Physiology quiz item #1:
I love the last letter of the alphabet

You might be surprised to learn that researchers have discovered a single treatment that boosts energy levels, improves memory, increases your ability to concentrate, strengthens the immune system, and decreases your risk of being killed in accidents. Sound too good to be true? It gets even better. If you knew the treatment was completely free, had no side effects, and that you would consider it highly enjoyable, would you try it? Sure, you would. The answer is an extra sixty to ninety minutes of sleep each night.[1] Perhaps you've been able to keep up with your modern, supercharged life by working all day, completing personal work and home chores late into the night, and sleeping an hour less than is optimal. Warning: without the proper sleep, you'll experience fatigue, lack of energy, difficulty concentrating, and irritability the next day. While the body can dig into its reserves for a few days, prolonged time of inadequate sleep is virtually guaranteed to reduce your effectiveness at anything you attempt to do.

In this chapter, you'll learn how to achieve quality, restful, undisturbed sleep. You'll find out when and if you should nap. You'll discover how your circadian rhythms are impacted by too much or not enough sleep. I'll show you how much sleep you need, how to achieve undisturbed sleep, and how to adopt proper sleep behaviors, so you feel refreshed and recharged in the morning, without becoming fatigued in the afternoon.

▼ ▼ ▼

As any parent of young children knows, sleep can be a fleeting thing the first few years. Sleep deprivation starts before the baby even arrives. But lack of sleep due to having children is a temporary inconvenience. However, lack of sleep over a long period of time is downright dangerous. In the short term, lack of sleep can have the following results:

- *Decreased performance and alertness:* Sleep deprivation induces significant reductions in performance and alertness. Reducing your nighttime sleep by as little as one and a half hours for just one night could result in a reduction of daytime alertness by as much as 32 percent.
- *Memory and cognitive impairment:* Decreased alertness and excessive daytime sleepiness impair your memory and your cognitive ability—your ability to think and process information.
- *Stress on relationships:* Disruption of a bed partner's sleep due to a sleep disorder may cause significant problems for the relationship (for example, separate bedrooms, conflicts, moodiness, and so forth).
- *Poor quality of life:* You might, for example, be unable to participate in certain activities that require sustained attention, like going to the movies, seeing your child in a school play, or watching a favorite TV show.
- *Lowered immune system:* Your body makes the most immune-strengthening repairs to your cells during the last,

longest period of REM sleep, which begins only after seven hours of slumber, says Philip Tierno, Ph.D., director of clinical microbiology and immunology at New York University Medical Center. A solid night of shut-eye will stave off illness.[2] A Harvard study reported in the journal *Neuron* (July 3, 2002) concurs: the final two hours of a full night's sleep are critical for the stage of sleep (stage 2 non–rapid eye movement, or NREM) that allows the maximum benefit for learning motor skills.

- *Occupational injury:* Excessive sleepiness also contributes to a greater than twofold higher risk of sustaining an occupational injury.

- *Automobile injury:* The National Highway Traffic Safety Administration (NHTSA) estimates conservatively that each year drowsy driving is responsible for at least 100,000 automobile crashes, 71,000 injuries, and 1,550 fatalities.[3]

- *Appetite:* According to the *Journal of the American Medical Association* and *Lancet,* sleep deprivation can negatively influence the stress hormone cortisol. If you aren't getting adequate sleep, you may be hungry even after eating a sufficient amount of food. In addition to affecting appetite control, sleep loss can also interfere with carbohydrate metabolism (the process of breaking down carbs), which leads to an increase in blood glucose levels, causing insulin to be released, which can lead to weight gain and increased fat storage.[4] Try this online test to see if you're sleep-deprived: http://www.smmc.com/Epworth-Sleepiness-Scale.105.0.html.

▲ ENERGY BOOSTER | **Get the right amount of sleep**

Tonight, you are going to get the proper amount of sleep—for you. Every individual is different. It's not too late to raise your personal energy level by getting the proper amount of sleep. Most people aged sixteen to sixty-five require six to nine hours per night, but you may need somewhere between five and ten. Don't be afraid to experiment until you get it right. To learn more about sleep deprivation and how to fight it, visit http://www.sleep-deprivation.com.

The common sleep wisdom has been to work eight hours, sleep eight hours, and rest eight hours. But some people need more sleep and some need less. Your exact sleep requirements depend on many factors:

- your age (infants, 16 hours; babies, 10–14 hours; young children, 10–12 hours; teenagers, 9 hours; adults, 7–8 hours),
- how much your parents slept (genetics),
- the type of work you do during waking hours,
- the amount of exercise you get,
- whether you're still growing,
- your sleep behaviors before bedtime,
- your stress level,
- how much caffeine, nicotine, and alcohol you consumed during the day,
- the quality of your sleep, and
- your body clock.

Try not to vary the hours when you go to bed and when you wake up, even on weekends. A consistent sleep schedule trains your body to go to sleep and wake up at set times. If you are getting enough sleep, meaning you're going to bed and waking up at about the same time each day without daytime sleepiness, you won't be able to sleep in on the weekend. If you sleep longer on weekends than you do during the week, you have a sleep debt. When you work, you drain your energy account. When you sleep, you replenish it. If your body needs eight hours of sleep, and you get only six each night during the week, you are a night of sleep behind come the weekend. Starting today, commit to going to bed on time to get the amount of sleep your body requires. How will you know? With the right amount of sleep, you will wake up feeling refreshed, full of energy, and will generally not get sleepy during the day. Not enough sleep will leave you sluggish, fuzzy-headed, and moody. Too much sleep will result in fragmented and shallow sleep. Sleep as much as needed to feel healthy the following day, but not more. Use this helpful sleep diary to track your progress: http://www.helpguide.org/life/sleep_diary.pdf.

▲ ▲ ▲
▼ ▼ ▼

▼ ENERGY BANDIT #2 | Too many cat naps

According to the American Academy of Sleep Medicine, you should try to avoid napping at all during the day if you have trouble sleeping at night (e.g., insomnia, disturbed sleep, or wakeful sleep), because short naps during the day can partially satisfy your body's need to sleep at night.[5] If you doze off while reading a book or watching television early in the evening, it may be harder for you to fall asleep at night. Without napping, when you're ready for sleep, you'll be truly exhausted, so you'll fall asleep more quickly and sleep more soundly.

▲ ENERGY BOOSTER | Nap wisely

If you don't have sleep problems and absolutely must take a nap, limit it to one hour and make sure you wake up before 3:00 PM. If you sleep more than sixty minutes, you risk experiencing sleep inertia, or grogginess, when you awake. You also want to make sure your nap is finished four to six hours before you retire for the evening, or it could affect your night's slumber. Mednick, Stickhold, and other Harvard researchers reported in *Nature Neuroscience* (July 2002) that a sixty-minute nap improved afternoon performance on learning tasks, in essence reversing the effects of information overload from earlier in the day. The slow-wave and REM sleep experienced in an hour-long nap refreshed the neural networks. An hour-long nap provided four times as much refreshing sleep as a half-hour nap. "This new linkage of naps to learning a repetitive task is exciting, but it's too soon to say that naps work like this for everybody," remarked psychologist Rosalind Cartwright of Rush-Presbyterian St. Luke's Medical Center in Chicago.

▲ ▲ ▲
▼ ▼ ▼

▼ ENERGY BANDIT #3 | Sleep disorders

Sleep deprivation could be due to an unrecognized sleep disorder. According to the National Institute of Neurological Disorders and Stroke, chronic, long-term sleep disorders affect at least 40 million Americans each year. Left untreated, sleep disorders, and the resulting sleep deprivation, will likely interfere with your work, driving, and social activities and have negative effects on your physical and mental well-being.[6]

More than one hundred sleep disorders exist, including sleep apnea, narcolepsy, insomnia, and restless legs syndrome. Sleep disorders are classified into three major categories: lack of sleep (e.g., insomnia), disturbed sleep (e.g., sleep apnea, REM sleep behavior disorder, restless legs syndrome, and periodic limb movement disorder), and excessive sleep (e.g., narcolepsy).[7]

In the long term, the clinical consequences of untreated sleep disorders are large indeed. Most individuals develop cognitive deficits from chronic sleep debt after only a few nights of reduced sleep quality or quantity, and new evidence suggests additional important health-related consequences from sleep debt, related, for example, to common viral illnesses, diabetes, obesity, heart disease, and depression. Findings from a recent study of young adult men placed on a restricted sleep schedule of four hours each night for six consecutive nights showed altered metabolism of glucose with an insulin-resistance pattern similar to that observed in elderly men. The implications from this study, if replicated, are that chronic sleep loss may contribute to obesity, diabetes, heart disease, and other age-related chronic disorders.[8]

Studies show an increased mortality risk for those reporting less than six or seven hours per night. One study found that reduced sleep time is a greater mortality risk than smoking, high blood pressure, and heart disease. Sleep disturbance is also one of the leading predictors of institutionalization in the elderly, and severe insomnia triples the mortality risk in elderly men.[9]

▲ ENERGY BOOSTER | **Get tested**

First, you want to rule out a sleeping disorder. Oh, sure, not you, right? Your irritability during the day? A grouchiness problem. Your sleepiness in the afternoon? A big lunch. Constantly tired? Too much work. Snoring? Your grandfather snored too. Before you know it, you're addicted to Red Bull, since coffee no longer gives you a kick. Sound like you? Sleep apnea is almost impossible to self-diagnose, because you are unconscious when it happens. If you experience any difficulty with sleep, including

- difficulty falling or staying asleep,
- loud snoring,
- difficulty staying awake during the daytime (excessive sleepiness),
- sleeping too much,
- difficulty sleeping during normal sleep hours at nighttime,
- abnormal behaviors during sleep that disrupt sleep, or
- unrefreshing sleep,

you might ask your primary-care physician to order an oximetry test, which measures the level of oxygen in your blood while you sleep, or a polysomnography test, which monitors brain waves, muscle tension, eye movement, respiration, oxygen level in the blood, and audio issues (such as snoring and gasping). If you're feeling tired during the day, rule out a medical sleeping problem first, and then treat the deprivation with behavioral changes. Medical disorders may be treated through mouth appliances, position therapy, surgery, or a CPAP (continuous positive airway pressure) machine.

If your body mass index (BMI) indicates that you are obese, weight loss is required for improved sleep. Your doctor will probably want you to complete a sleep diary. You can get a booklet through the American Academy of Sleep Medicine (www.aasmnet.org).

▲ ▲ ▲
▼ ▼ ▼

▼ ENERGY BANDIT #4 | Obesity

Significant weight loss can improve the sleep patterns of severely obese people, leading to less daytime sleepiness and better quality of life, a study by the Monash University Centre of Obesity Research and Education has found.[10]

▲ ENERGY BOOSTER | Lose weight

Overweight people are especially at risk for obstructive sleep apnea, or OSA, which is a sleep-related breathing disorder that causes your body to stop breathing during sleep. OSA occurs when the tissue in the back of the throat collapses and blocks the airway, which keeps air from getting into the lungs. Up to 48 percent of obese men and 38 percent of obese women suffer from OSA. Your neck gets thicker as you gain weight, which increases the level of fat in the back of the throat, narrowing the airway. With more fat in the throat, your airway is more likely to be blocked. People with a neck size of more than seventeen inches have a higher incidence of OSA. Many people with OSA also have high blood pressure.[11]

Interestingly enough, obesity and sleep is a vicious cycle, because a Columbia University study showed that not getting enough sleep puts you at increased risk for weight gain! Out of eighteen thousand adults, those who slept less than four hours per night were 73 percent more likely to be obese than those who slept seven to nine hours; five hours decreased it to 50 percent; six hours decreased it even more to 23 percent.[12] Scientists believe a lack of sleep lowers your leptin level, which is a protein that tells your brain when your stomach is full.

Researchers at the University of Chicago (*The Journal of the American Medical Association,* August 16, 2000) also found a link between weight gain in men and age. The male brain produces and secretes growth hormones—an important part of the body's weight regulation system—during deep or slow-wave sleep (not during rapid eye movement, or REM sleep, when dreaming occurs and brain waves are moving faster). But as men age, they get less and less deep sleep. Researchers found that by age forty-five, men have nearly lost the ability to fall into deep sleep. As a result, growth hormone production falls, and the fight against flab begins. Since there's nothing you can do about aging, men must monitor their diets more carefully after age forty-five.

▲ ▲ ▲
▼ ▼ ▼

▼ ENERGY BANDIT #5 | **Faulty circadian rhythms**

Circadian is Latin for "about a day." You've heard the terms "body clock," "biological clock," "master clock," or the "circadian rhythm," which are all the same thing—a specific area of the brain called the hypothalamus, which controls your activity, energy, and how well you feel. The body clock sends out the signals that change the level of hormones and neurotransmitters during the twenty-four-hour day. It also regulates things like hormones, body temperature, and heart activity and is responsible for regulating bodily functions that specifically relate to the timing of sleep, called the sleep/wake cycle. The biological sleep clock is triggered by sunlight and darkness. Usually the biological clock and the real world clock are the same; when they are not the same, sleep problems result. If you work late-night shifts or travel internationally to reverse time zones, you will often experience a disruption of your sleep/wake cycle and feel sleepy. Or if it is 10:00 PM real time, but your body feels like it is 8:00, you won't get sleepy until very late at night. But if you go to bed at midnight and have to get up at 6:30 AM for a meeting, you're going to be sleepy during the day. Conversely, if it's 8:00 PM, but your body clock says it's 10:00 PM, you're going to be sleepy and perhaps doze in front of the television, and then wonder why, at midnight, you can't sleep. You actually got some of your sleep earlier in the evening, and now you have insomnia.

▲ ENERGY BOOSTER | **Reset your body clock**

Sometimes the problem is a body clock that's out of whack. Delayed circadian disorder (DCR) means your circadian rhythms are running slower than a normal twenty-four-hour period, which means you're producing the wrong type of hormones at the wrong time of day. Because your cycle is too slow, your pineal gland releases the nighttime hormone melatonin too late, often causing you to fall asleep later. When you need to get up, your body clock may think it is 3:00 AM, so it takes you several hours to produce serotonin and feel active and energetic.

One common cause is seasonal affective disorder (SAD). This is a form of depression that affects a half million people in the United

States; another 10 to 20 percent of the population may experience mild SAD. It is more common in northern geographic areas where there is a more dramatic lack of sunlight in winter. SAD is accompanied by a drop in energy level, weight gain, fatigue, and difficulty concentrating.[13] It usually begins in late fall or early winter and lasts until early summer, and is related to a lack of natural sunlight. Not only is it more cloudy in winter, but you may venture outdoors less frequently due to rain or drastic cold.

I went through a strange bout of insomnia a few years ago, which was abnormal for me, and went to talk with my doctor about it. It was during the cold winter months of Denver. I was feeling a bit blue and having difficulty getting started in the morning. He said those were symptoms of SAD, and rather than putting me on medication, he suggested that perhaps I should consider light treatment for a few months. Because it was winter, perhaps my body clock wasn't receiving the right sunlight signals, which tell your brain to "wake up." After a bit of research, I purchased an Apollo goLITE (www.mygolite .com), which uses the Bluewave technology discovered in 1986 by the National Institutes of Health. Bluewave is about twenty times brighter than natural light and safely resets your body clock when used correctly. I took a quiz on the Web site and followed the instructions based upon my results, which for me was thirty minutes a day of light treatment at 7:30 AM. As my circadian rhythms began to normalize, I noticed improved energy during the day and the ability to fall asleep and wake up more easily.

If you're having chronic sleep problems, schedule an appointment with your doctor today to discuss it. Use medication as a *last* resort. Some sleep medications, such as Rozerem, Ambien, and Sonota, can adjust the sleep/wake cycle and make your body feel like it's time to sleep when it normally wouldn't. Some doctors prescribe sleep medicine as a temporary "fix" when insomnia kicks in from stress or illness. The most significant concern about the use of medications for treating insomnia is that medication does not address the root cause of the problem, and instead becomes a crutch to lean on rather than a cure. Just as you would not leave a cast on a broken bone indefinitely because it would cause the muscle to atrophy, sleep medication should be seen as a temporary aid for sleep problems and not a long-term one. Bottom line: don't go straight to medication if you are having sleep problems. Try the behavioral changes outlined in this chapter first, to make sure you're doing everything possible to help your body sleep.

▲ ▲ ▲
▼ ▼ ▼

▼ ENERGY BANDIT #6 | Poor sleep behaviors

If you do anything stimulating right before bed—such as arguing with your spouse, exercising, or watching a horror movie—you will have a harder time shutting down and going to sleep. Or perhaps your spouse snores like mine does. Don't just suffer—deal with it. I sleep with earplugs (I like www.hearos.com), which drown out snoring and other background noise but still allow me to hear my alarm clock. If you're disturbed by passing airplanes, neighbors, or other noises, you may also want to consider earplugs. Perhaps you're too hot or too cold (an ideal sleeping temperature is no less than 68 degrees and no higher than 72 degrees), or your pets wake you up at night. Make a concerted effort to determine why you're sleeping poorly and commit yourself to changing your behavior where you can.

▲ ENERGY BOOSTER | Create the right sleeping environment

When you lie down, can you fall asleep within a matter of minutes? No? Then you might not have the right mental association to your bed. When you get into your bed, your brain should tell your body to shut down and go to sleep. Unfortunately, many people crawl into bed and don't put their heads on the pillow. They eat. They watch television. They read. They do paperwork. They have conversations with their significant other. They worry. As a result, these associations encourage wakefulness, and the brain soon disassociates the bed with sleep. When you finally tell it, "Okay, I'm serious now," it takes longer to get the message. Use your bed only for sleeping and intimate relations with your significant other. Eating, watching television, reading, working on your computer, and any other activity should be done out of bed, preferably in a completely different room. Your bedroom should be your sleeping sanctuary—a place where your mind automatically goes to sleep. You're better off doing something relaxing an hour before bedtime, such as a warm bath, aromatherapy, knitting, petting your cat, doing dishes, or reading.

▼ ENERGY BANDIT #7 | Eating and drinking at the wrong times

Digestion usually takes several hours, so rethink mealtime according to your bedtime. Digesting food takes a lot of energy and distracts your body from sleep.

▲ ENERGY BOOSTER | Eat and drink to sleep

Elizabeth L. Vliet, M.D., author of *It's My Ovaries, Stupid!*, says to take 200 to 400 mg of magnesium and 500 mg of calcium thirty to sixty minutes before bedtime to help your body prepare for sleep. "Studies show that your brain needs adequate levels of these vitamins, along with optimal levels of estradiol, in order to regulate sleep," says Vliet. Avoid eating a large meal just before bedtime; however, don't go to bed ravenous—it's about balance—have a light snack if you must. Michael Breus, Ph.D., of SoundSleep Solutions, says, "milk, tuna, halibut, pumpkin, artichokes, avocados, almonds, eggs, peaches, walnuts, apricots, oats, asparagus, potatoes, and bananas" all promote good sleep. Also watch your alcohol consumption before bedtime. Alcohol can indeed make you sleepy, but it is considered a stimulant and will cause wakeful sleep, nightmares, sweats, and headaches as your body clears it from your system. Try warm milk instead or even a Benadryl if you're desperate. If you want to avoid midnight trips to the bathroom, stop drinking large amounts early in the evening. I go to bed at 10:00, and I stop drinking at 7:00. If I'm thirsty, I take a *small* sip of water.

▲ ▲ ▲
▼ ▼ ▼

▼ ENERGY BANDIT #8 | You don't sleep well when you travel

While airline travel is a necessity for most business travelers and a convenience for leisure travelers, it is fraught with its own disadvantages. After traveling across several time zones, you may experience insomnia, irritability, dehydration, a loss of coordination, and a general lack of energy, collectively known as jet lag, which throws off your regular body clock. Severe cases last several days and can affect your performance and ability to concentrate. To circumvent these side effects, you must put some advance thought and planning into travel.

▲ ENERGY BOOSTER | Protect your sleep when you travel

I love staying at Crowne Plaza hotels (www.crowneplaza.com) because they understand the need for great sleep. When you enter your room, you'll find a small package on your bed containing earplugs, eye mask, lavender aromatherapy spray, and a sleep CD with advice and sounds conducive to sleep, based on advice from Breus.

The best parts of the package are the drape clip to keep out unwanted light and a night-light to provide soft lighting on the way to the bathroom. After a long day of client meetings and presentations, it's nice to get back to the hotel and enjoy the sleep package, a bed with a thick duvet, and a mattress without any body impressions— almost worth being away from home for, but not quite.

If you are traveling to a location with a drastic time-zone difference, try resetting your body clock several days in advance. Wake up, eat, and go to bed earlier or later, depending upon your goal, until you approximate the day-night pattern you'll be adapting to at your destination. Some globe-trotters have told me they even reset their watches to the destination time, so they can make the psychological switch as well. Try to get additional sleep before leaving and during your flight. Avoid alcohol (two alcoholic drinks consumed in a pressurized cabin have the physical effect of four drinks at sea level), caffeine, and high-calorie meals. Try to arrive a day earlier than necessary, so that your brain can make adjustments before you're expected to be coherent. In general, allow for about a day on either end to let your body adjust.

▲ ▲ ▲

Two

Diet

Have you ever said, "I don't have time to eat properly"? You rationalize poor eating habits, saying your busy schedule doesn't give you the ability to make the right eating choices. Plus, you crave bad foods, partly because you're stressed out, run-down, and not getting enough sleep, which can leave you wanting carbohydrates.

Obviously, balanced meals and nutritious foods are required for high energy. When you eat balanced meals, including the right amounts of protein and complex carbohydrates, your body receives the protein, fiber, vitamins, minerals, and phytochemicals (such as beta-carotene) it needs. You need to eat a diet that includes whole grains, colorful fruits and vegetables, proteins, and heart-healthy fats. This is a fantastic time to be on a program for healthier eating. The food industry is finally responding to the trans-fats issue and is actually using more whole grains. This chapter is about how you can make simple changes in your daily choices that can make a big difference in your energy level.

▼ ▼ ▼

▼ ENERGY BANDIT #1 | Consuming too many calories

Being overweight has myriad health consequences, not least of which is low energy. Poor diet and physical inactivity, resulting in an energy imbalance (more calories consumed than expended), are the most important factors contributing to the increase in the numbers of overweight and obese people in America. Moreover, being overweight and being obese are major risk factors for certain chronic diseases, such as diabetes.

▲ ENERGY BOOSTER | Make sure you're eating the right amount of food—and no more

If you eat too much and move too little, you will gain weight. If you want to lose weight, do the reverse. But if you don't know how much you're eating during the day, how many calories certain foods have, and how much you should eat for weight gain, loss, or maintenance, you won't likely guess correctly. But one size does not fit all.

Caloric intake depends upon age, gender, weight, activity level, and whether you're trying to gain, maintain, or lose weight. For example, the average man needs nearly 35 percent more calories per day than the average woman. There is a daily calorie requirements calculator at http://www.cancer.org/docroot/PED/content/PED_6_1x_Calorie_Calculator.asp, where you can find out the number of calories you need to maintain your current weight.

One way to know if you've been eating too many calories, too few, or just the right amount is to calculate your body mass index (BMI):

1. First take your height in inches. For example, I'm 5 feet 5 inches, which equals 65 inches.

2. Then multiply your height in inches by itself. So 65 × 65 = 4,225.

3. Now take your weight (I'm 138 pounds currently) and divide it by the figure above. So 138 ÷ 4,225 = .03266 (you can round to 5 figures).

4. Then multiply that number by 703. So .03266 × 703 = 22.9, which reflects my current BMI.

You can also calculate your BMI at http://www.bcm.edu/cnrc/caloriesneed.htm. What does your resulting number mean?

18.5 = underweight
18.5–24.9 = normal weight
25–29.9 = overweight
>30 = obese

BMI isn't foolproof, however; if you're athletic, for example, your extra muscle, which is heavier than fat, may throw off your numbers. So another way to determine whether you're eating too many calories is to get out your measuring tape and measure around your middle. Extra fat in our belly area may put our health at risk, even if we are at a healthy weight. Men who have a waist size greater than forty inches and women who have a waist size greater than thirty-five inches are at a higher risk of diabetes, problems with cholesterol and triglycerides, high blood pressure, and heart disease because of excess abdominal fat.[1]

Consider losing weight if your BMI indicates you are overweight or obese. Here are some ideas for shedding the pounds:

- Aim to cut 500 calories per day, which amounts to one pound per week or two (depending on your level of activity and how efficiently you metabolize calories).

- If it's in a box, don't eat it. If it doesn't occur naturally, don't eat it. Eat lots of vitamin-rich fruits and vegetables and proteins, which are more satiating than carbs and fats.
- Eat slowly. It takes a long time (approximately twenty minutes) for your brain to receive the "full" signal. If you're eating out, leave the restaurant and go somewhere else for dessert. Chances are, by the time you get there, you won't want it.
- Try cooking healthy dishes with exotic flavor boosters like wasabi, pomegranate molasses, or tandoori paste, which have little or no fat.
- Read the labels. Avoid foods with high-fructose corn syrup or trans fats (or the tip-off: partially hydrogenated oil). Also watch the serving suggestions carefully: a snack-sized bag of 150-calories-per-serving Cheez Doodles is actually two servings. Listing sugar in several different forms (dextrose, honey, and evaporated cane juice, to name just three) is a trick that manufacturers use to push it down the ingredients list.
- Be mindful of the big cost of little bites. A handful of candy corn, the top of a muffin, a bite of your child's bagel with strawberry cream cheese, one spoonful of Häagen-Dazs, and a few French fries from your spouse's plate can amount to hundreds more calories each day. Resist the urge to pop one more little thing into your mouth. Or if you do eat this way, be sure to include the calories in your overall daily eating plan.
- Don't eat while you're doing other activities. Reserve mealtimes for simply eating—at the table—with no television, computer, or reading materials to distract you from what's going into your mouth. Watching television while munching, viewing a movie at the theater with a big tub of popcorn, or reading the paper while eating cinnamon rolls are sure recipes for disaster. Slow down, focus on the food in front of you, and stop when you are full.

- Avoid combination foods: stuffed-crust pizza, cheese fries, fried ice cream, and peanut-butter-packed pretzels . . . or my son James's favorite—a Dairy Queen Brownie Earthquake (740 calories). By combining several of your favorite things, it takes what was already an indulgence into the stratosphere.

- Don't cut out *all* fat. Research by Dr. Steven Clinton at the Ohio State University Comprehensive Cancer Center in Columbus showed that certain vitamins and cancer-fighting compounds, such as lycopene and beta-carotene in vegetables, are "fat soluble." That means some fat must be present for the body to absorb the nutrients. So if you skip the avocado or cheese in your dish to save calories, you aren't reaping the full benefits of the vegetables.

- Once you do lose weight, your newly lean body will require fewer calories than it did pre-diet. You'll need to eat at lower levels since your baseline caloric need has shifted downward.

- Eat breakfast. A study of people in the National Weight Control Registry (more than six thousand people who lost an average of sixty-seven pounds and kept it off for at least six years) found that if they ate a morning meal, "they were better able to control their food intake all day long," explains James O. Hill, Ph.D., *Shape* magazine advisory board member and director of the Center for Human Nutrition at the University of Colorado.

- Eat, don't drink, your calories; avoid that morning Starbucks latte, sweetened iced tea, regular cola, and fruit juices, which aren't as filling as whole foods and add unnecessary calories.

- Brush your teeth after every meal. Yes, it's good for your teeth. More important, the fresh minty taste in your mouth can be a cue to stop eating and thwart your desire to dip into the spaghetti again.

▲ ▲ ▲

▼ ▼ ▼

| **Eating an unbalanced diet**

Have you ever tried one of those "fad" diets like eating nothing but lettuce and grapefruit, or drinking only a lemon-and-cayenne-pepper mixture for five days? I'm sure you lost weight, but your energy was probably in the basement from lack of nourishment.

▲ ENERGY BOOSTER | **A fad diet is not the answer; a balanced diet is**

The best weight-loss plan is also the one that's the most nutritious on a consistent basis. A 2004 study conducted by the Weight Control and Diabetes Research Center at Brown Medical School confirms that eating consistently aids weight management. The research studied fourteen hundred people from the National Weight Control Registry. It showed that people who ate consistent amounts (versus more on some days and less on others) were 1.5 times more likely to maintain their weight.[2] So stop talking about diets and start thinking like a healthy person. You can't be overweight if you don't behave overweight.

You can't survive on meat alone, bread alone, or pie alone. For the best quality of life, you need your carbs, proteins, and fats. The best diet is high protein, low fat, high fiber, low sodium, with fruits and vegetables, which are antioxidants. This will lessen the possibility of disease, keep the weight off, give the body more energy, and make you look and feel like a new person. The benefits of these foods are important. The body needs them all. There is not one that is more important than another.

What food should you include in your diet every day for a balanced, consistent diet? Divide your daily diet into seven main areas[3]:

1. **Grains (carbohydrates)** give your body fiber to aid digestion; carbohydrates to provide energy; iron to carry oxygen; and vitamin B to help use energy in your body. Carbohydrates provide fuel for your body. There are two forms of carbohydrates: complex carbs (starches) and simple carbs (sugars). Sugar offers a quick boost and starches offer a longer boost. Therefore, your carbohydrates should mostly come from complex carbs such as fruits, grains, legumes, starches, and vegetables, because they keep your energy up longer and also contain vitamins, minerals, and other nutrients—a bonus. Avoid simple carbs—sugar in the form of processed cakes, candy, and cookies—which will spike your energy and then drop you even lower. Complex carbs are a key factor in weight management. The digestive system uses up more energy in metabolizing starches than it does in metabolizing fat. These complex carbs are also good at recognizing when enough food has been consumed and signals our bodies when we are full.

2. **Vegetables** give us vitamin A to help vision and vitamin C to help with the healing process and fight infection; fiber to aid in digestion; iron for muscle/nerve function; magnesium for carrying oxygen in red blood cells and muscle; and folic acid to aid in growth and cell division. Try to eat a variety of veggies with different colors (green, orange, yellow, and red) to ensure that you're getting a range of healthy nutrients.

3. **Fruits** give your body vitamin A; vitamin C; fiber to help digest food; folic acid to aid in growth and cell division; and potassium to maintain heartbeat, regulate fluid, and aid in muscle function. You can eat them frozen, canned, or dried (avoid juice), but fresh is best.

4. **Meat and beans** give us protein to aid muscle growth; vitamin B to help us use energy; and iron to carry oxygen.

Proteins are essential for strong muscles, bones, teeth, fingernails, and hair growth. Proteins build and rebuild tissue in the body and regulate chemical functions. Every cell has protein. Protein also aids in growth, maintenance, and resisting infection. The best forms of protein are complete proteins, which are essential amino acids. Pick lean cuts of meat. Strive to eat fish twice a week.

5. **Milk and dairy.** Proteins are also contained in dairy products (milk, yogurt, cheese, and eggs), meat, grains, wheat germ, nuts, and soy. Milk also gives your body calcium to maintain bones and teeth; protein to help with growth and maintenance of body tissue; riboflayin to help the body use energy; and calcium to strengthen your bones and lower your risk of osteoporosis.

6. **Oils.** Fats can be good or bad. Our bodies require good fats— such as those found in avocados, raw nuts, cold-water fish (salmon, trout, and tuna), and oils (olive, sesame, and sunflower)—as they aid in storing energy, maintaining healthy skin and hair, providing essential fatty acids, and telling the body when it is full and satisfied. These fats also carry fat-soluble vitamins such as A, D, E, and K. Bad fats—such as trans fats or partially hydrogenated vegetable oils—cause the body higher levels of the fat-storage hormone insulin. Limit fats that are high in saturated fat (solid at room temperature), such as butter or lard.

7. **Discretionary calories** come from any fun food or treat you want.

▲ ▲ ▲

▼ ▼ ▼

▼ ENERGY BANDIT #3 | A poor eating schedule

Eating randomly throughout the day or evening can prevent you from getting a handle on just how much you're actually consuming.

▲ ENERGY BOOSTER | Keep track of your eating patterns

For a great food diary to log your food intake, visit www.self.com/goal. Or perhaps there are key times of the day when you know you overeat. Maybe it's right when you get home, during the afternoon slump at work, or once you get the kids to bed. Perhaps it's when you plop down in front of the television. Identify the target time, place, activity, people, and moods that trigger the impulse to eat junk food, eat too fast, or overeat. Then come up with an alternate activity to replace eating. Fold laundry in front of the television to keep your hands busy. Or switch to low-cal, air-popped popcorn. My problem is nighttime snacking. I tend to do well during the day, because I stay busy and productive, but then I slide in the evenings, often indulging in one too many snacks or treats. It's helpful to set up an eating schedule around the key times you're more likely to have problems. I decided that I needed to have all my food eaten by 7:00 and would plan an activity that's incompatible with eating, such as walking my dog, playing a board game with the kids, or taking a bath. This plan has made a nice difference for me.

▲ ▲ ▲

▼ ▼ ▼

▼ ENERGY BANDIT #4 | Not following a customized food plan

The reason most people hate tracking their food intake is because trying to gauge calories can get complicated. But here's the good news: you do *not* have to know the calorie count of every food you ingest to eat the proper amounts of food each day—you need to know only the serving size for each food.

▲ ENERGY BOOSTER | Create a customized eating plan

Each person, based on gender, calorie requirement, exercise level, weight loss goal, and so forth, has to put together his or her own eating plan. I try to consume around 1,800 calories a day right now (female, 138 pounds, moderate activity, slight weight-loss plan). So my intake usually includes the following:

- Grains: 5 servings—about 80 calories per serving—400 total calories
- Vegetables: 4 servings—about 25 calories per serving—100 total calories
- Fruits: 3 servings—about 60 calories per serving—180 total calories
- Milk: 2½ servings—about 100 calories per serving—250 total calories
- Meat and beans: 3 servings—150 to 170 calories per serving—up to 510 total calories
- Oils: 5 servings—about 45 calories per serving—225 total calories
- Discretionary calories: 140 calories of anything

You can get a calorie count and suggested food-group intake tailored for you at the U.S. Department of Agriculture Web site, www.mypyramid.org, where you can enter your age, gender, and activity level. You can download a nifty PDF card of serving sizes for the different food groups from the National Institutes of Health to cut out and keep on your refrigerator at http://hp2010.nhlbihin.net/portion/servingcard7.pdf. For a free calorie counter, go to http://www.caloriesperhour.com/. For expanded food lists, calorie counts, and sample menus, go to www.self.com/goal.

Or you can estimate serving size by picturing the following:

Food item	Serving size	Picture for serving size
Bread	1 slice	Audio cassette tape
Rice	1 cup	Tennis ball
Salad greens	1 cup	Baseball
Tomato juice	¾ cup	Small Styrofoam cup
Cooked broccoli	1/2 cup	Scoop of ice cream
Grapes	1/2 cup (15)	Lightbulb
Apple or orange	1 piece	Tennis ball
Peanut butter	1 tablespoon	Ping-Pong ball
Cooked meat, fish, poultry	3 ounces	Deck of cards
Cheese	1 ounce	Pair of dice
Ice cream	1 cup	Baseball
Butter	1 teaspoon	Postage stamp
Salad dressing	2 tablespoons	Ping-Pong ball

(*Bonus:* Send an e-mail to Servings@The Productivity Pro.com and receive a sample serving-size chart showing the food groups, calories, serving sizes, and food choices for a 1,700-calorie diet. Modify it to fit your needs and chart your food intake each day.)

▲ ▲ ▲

▼ ▼ ▼

Eating more than the recommended serving size

How much should you eat of each food? If you're like many people, you're eating too many oils and discretionary calories and not enough of the other categories. "Studies have shown that the bigger the portion, the more people eat," said Barbara Rolls, Ph.D., professor of nutritional sciences at Penn State University and author of *The Volumetrics Eating Plan* (Morrow Cookbooks, 2005). A study headed up by Rolls and published in *Obesity* (2004, volume 12: pages 562–568) researched what would happen when customers in a public restaurant were served differing sizes of baked ziti, which varied between a standard portion and a larger serving containing 50 percent more food (the price was the same). The results showed that even when customers were served 50 percent more ziti, they still ate nearly all of it, or an average of 172 additional calories! Surprisingly, they also ate more of the accompaniments as well. When rating the size of the portion after the meal, diners rated the size of each portion as equally appropriate.[4] This study just goes to show that we can't count on other people to know the correct serving size. We have to be knowledgeable about what's on our plates.

If you went to a restaurant and ordered pancakes and were served one solitary pancake, you might think, "That's all?" One pancake is one serving—you could have three pancakes, but you have to count three servings of grains. If you need five servings of grains a day, you have only two left for the entire day. So a "serving" is not the amount you're expected to eat in one sitting. It takes you all day to reach your daily allowance in each food group. Servings are simply building blocks to help you put together a healthy, balanced meal each day.

Another potential contributor to the postprandial energy crash is something called the "satiety reflex." The scenario goes like this:

when your stomach is filled, your thyroid secretes a hormone called calcitonin. This is a chemical signal that tells your brain to stop eating and go to sleep, because sleeping can aid digestion.

▲ ENERGY BOOSTER | **Cut back on portion sizes**

Losing weight can be difficult in our supersized culture. Here are a few ways to keep you from polishing off too much food:

- Change your dinnerware to reflect correct portions. Use a ten-inch salad plate for your meal instead of a regular sixteen-inch dinner plate.
- Drink out of tall, thin glasses like flutes.
- When you order at a restaurant, before the server even leaves your table, ask for half of your meal to be boxed when it's brought out. Most restaurant portions are much bigger than a regular meal serving. Now you automatically have a lunch to bring to work the next day.
- Eat a salad before your meal. A study at Penn State University found that subjects consumed 12 percent fewer calories during a meal when they ate a first-course salad than when they did not.
- When eating at a restaurant, share with your dining partner. Order one meal and ask the waitstaff to split it for you in the kitchen. Or order an appetizer or side dish as your meal, which is normally the right serving size.

▲ ▲ ▲

▼ ▼ ▼

▼ ENERGY BANDIT #6 | Not knowing "good" foods from "bad"

My heavens—good carbs, bad fat, lean protein—who can keep it all straight? Let me try to simplify things for you with a simple back-to-basics guide on how to eat to be at the correct weight for you and energized, without confusion or forbidden foods.

▲ ENERGY BOOSTER | Make better choices

Here's the skinny on food and energy:

Group	Select these foods if possible	Over these foods
Grains	Brown rice	Bagels
	Whole-wheat bread	Pastries
	Whole-wheat pasta	Doughnuts
	Cereal with 4 grams of fiber per serving	Sweetened cereal
	Sweet potatoes	White bread
Vegetables	Carrots	Broccoli with cheese sauce
	Broccoli	Packed vegetables with sauces
	Cauliflower	Creamed vegetables
	Squash	Avocado (extra fat, but healthy)
	Green beans	Olives (extra fat, but healthy)
	Peppers	Corn (a starch)

Group	Select these foods if possible	Over these foods
Fruits	Bananas	Sweetened fruit juices
	Apples	Canned fruit in syrup
	Oranges	Dried fruit (calorie-dense)
Milk	Skim milk	Eggnog
	Part-skim cottage cheese	Ice cream
	Carb-control yogurt	Whole milk
	Plain nonfat yogurt	Creamer
	Part-skim string or hard cheese	
Meat and Beans	Beans	Polish sausage
	Eggs	Bologna
	Skinless poultry	Marbled beef
	Lean cuts of beef	Hot dogs
	Tuna, cod, flounder	Bacon
	Scallops, clams, crab, mussels	Peanut butter
Oils	Fat-free mayonnaise	Mayonnaise
	Fat-free, low-sugar salad dressing	Miracle Whip
	Fats that are liquid at room temperature	Salad dressing
		Fats that are solid at room temperature
	Yogurt	Sour cream
	Applesauce	

Group	Select these foods if possible	Over these foods
Discretionary	Sugar-free Jell-O snack cups	Oreos
	Fat-free, sugar-free pudding	Doughnuts
	No-sugar-added Fudgsicles or Popsicles	Sugar candy
		Chocolate

For another great list of alternatives, check out http://www.health.gov/dietaryguidelines/dga2005/healthieryou/html/tips_healthy_subs.html.

▼ ENERGY BANDIT #7 | **Being unprepared for difficult food situations**

The workplace is filled with myriad food-related temptations. Betty Sue baked her homemade Christmas cookies with the sparkling colored sugar; you have a three-day conference where high-carb, high-fat meals are served and protein will be scarce; breakfast in a meeting usually consists of pastries and bagels; the company holiday party or potluck is right around the corner; your office has a party every month for people celebrating birthdays.

▲ ENERGY BOOSTER | **Plan in advance**

Luckily, you can still eat in moderation with a little bit of advance planning. Look ahead at your schedule and think about where you're going to be and what you'll need for the following tricky food situations:

- Bring something healthy if everyone is contributing to a potluck, so you will at least have something you like and can eat without guilt (hummus, salad, or a fresh fruit or vegetable plate are all good bets).
- If you have a holiday party you must attend, watch your food intake during the rest of the day. Go light that day to "save up" your calories for the special event. Just make sure you don't make a regular habit of this. You should still eat a light breakfast and lunch, however, because skipping food entirely will leave you ravenous and cause you to overeat.
- Cornell University researchers found that people who placed only two things on their plates at once served themselves 21 percent less food and made one less trip to the line, as compared with those who piled on a variety of foods.[5]
- If you have a cafeteria at work, you might get lazy preparing food at home, knowing you can always go there in a pinch. If you have a microwave available, bring something from home instead. If you pack it the night before, you won't have to stress in the morning while trying to get out the door.
- Before you go back to work on Monday, map out your meals for the week. Buy some quick-prep options, such as a stir-fry of precut veggies and cooked chicken strips. Always keep a bag of prewashed salad greens on hand. Look for ready-to-eat vegetables and precut fruits. Meals cooked at home tend to be higher in nutrients and lower in calories than take-out or eat-out.
- If you won't be home until late because you're out on the road visiting customers, then map out your route and figure out what restaurants you'll pass. Check out their menus on-line and be prepared for the healthy food you're going to or-

der before you arrive. Better yet, call in your order in advance so there's no wavering.

- If you know a meeting is going to run late one evening and you won't have time to cook, prepare a double recipe on another evening and freeze the leftovers. If you're flying, purchase healthy snacks for the plane before you board. When you're hungry, even airline food looks good.

- When traveling in a strange town, you may be forced to enter the fast-food drive-through lane. You don't have to blow your entire eating plan if you're careful. Panda Express, Chipotle, and Heidi's Brooklyn Deli are some local fast-food joints with healthy options. If you can't find the best choice, make a better food choice. It may not be the ideal one, but it's better than abandoning ship. Dr. Jo (a.k.a. Joanne V. Lichten, Ph.D.) says on AOL Diet and Fitness, "Fast food can fit into any diet." Dr. Jo says shrimp with garlic sauce, chicken fajitas, vegetarian pizza, Subway's sweet onion chicken teriyaki, and Wendy's Mandarin Chicken salad will all do nicely in a pinch.[6]

▲ ▲ ▲
▼ ▼ ▼

▼ ENERGY BANDIT #8 | Poor self-talk

I can just hear my mother saying, "Eat everything on your plate, because the poor children in China are starving!" Maybe your parents spoke of the poor, starving children in Africa or Ethiopia; regardless, many of us have heard a similar phrase uttered. Did you ever want to say, "Well, then put it in the mail and ship it to them"? Even then, as a child, I knew that admonishment was ridiculous. Forcing yourself to eat everything in front of you doesn't aid people in developing countries; it only hurts *you*. That would be like buying medicine when you have a cold, using half the package, and forcing yourself to take the rest of it even when you feel better.

▲ ENERGY BOOSTER | **Stop any counterproductive thinking**

What are the ingrained thoughts that go round in your mind and affect the way you eat? Many of them are learned from your family and culture and have been a part of your life forever, so they seem normal. If some of these thoughts sound familiar, resolve to replace them with healthier alternatives:

- "Always leave one bite of food on your plate, so people don't think you're a pig." If you have the correct serving size, you don't have to worry about consuming the entire portion.
- "Never refuse food from the host or hostess in someone's home." It is acceptable to decline a second serving, explaining that you're full and don't like to eat when you're not hungry.
- "You've already spoiled your diet today; you might as well eat a piece of cheesecake." If you've already consumed an extra 500 calories today, another 500 is not going to help.
- "It is dinnertime, and I'm not really hungry, but I guess I should eat." Use your own body clock to determine when to eat. Do not eat just because the kitchen clock says "it's time." You will know when it's time when you feel a gnawing in your stomach. Be careful not to confuse thirst, loneliness, or boredom with hunger.
- "If I don't want to gain weight, I can't have any dessert." Forbidding certain foods is a sure way to want more of them. To gain a pound, you must ingest an extra 3,500 calories. A Krispy Kreme glazed donut (my favorite) is 200 calories, far from derailing your entire diet. Just eat it purposefully and

savor every bite, taking the calories into account with your overall plans. Foods like doughnuts, cookies, or cake won't cause weight gain if you learn how to fit them in and eat them in moderation. So now I pair my doughnut with a leafy green salad and tuna and have at it!

▲ ▲ ▲

Three

Nutrition

Physiology quiz item #3:
Is sugar a nutrient?

Poor nutrition can be as draining as the wrong diet, and the consequences can sneak up on you. A friend of mine once went through a period in which she had low energy during the day, and she had to lie down frequently due to constant headaches. She just assumed that she had migraines and couldn't do much about it. Worried, her husband convinced her to go to the doctor for a physical, and after a series of tests, she was diagnosed with low iron content in her bloodstream. After receiving proper treatment, she felt better within a matter of weeks.

Sometimes, all you have to do to up your energy is to recognize the symptoms of nutritional imbalances, and then take steps to address them. Chapter 2 dealt with the food you eat; this chapter will deal with how nutrients are used by your body. In this chapter, you'll learn how your body uses that food for repair, growth, and energy. You'll discover the roles various nutrients have in maintaining health, and how to counter low energy with vitamins, water, and supplements. We'll also explore any poor nutrition habits and their impact on your energy, and I'll offer you options to help you overcome those problems.

▼ ▼ ▼

▼ ENERGY BANDIT #1 | **Nutrient deficiencies**

Under most circumstances, the human body is a marvelously well-balanced organic machine, but things can go wrong if you don't make sure that it gets all the special fuels and building materials it needs to function optimally. Unfortunately, the body can't synthesize some essential nutrients, so it has to obtain them from outside, usually as components of various foods.

▲ ENERGY BOOSTER | **Get a good balance of the essential nutrients**

It's amazing how many nutrients your body needs. Aside from the water, carbohydrates, proteins, and fats that comprise most of your daily intake, essential nutrients fall into four broad categories:

1. Fatty acids
2. Amino acids
3. Vitamins
4. Minerals

Recently many so-called "micronutrients" also have been recognized as necessary for good health. The problem is, no one quite agrees on exactly what these essential nutrients *are*. Estimates range from fifteen to ninety essential nutrients, depending on who's trying to sell what. I've summarized the ones that can affect your energy, some common sources, and the Recommended Daily Allowances (RDAs) of each below. Check your symptoms and eat more of what you might be lacking.

Nutrient	Function(s)	Deficiency Symptoms	Food Sources	RDA[1]
Essential fatty acids[2]				
Linolenic acid	Blood pressure regulation, clotting	Low energy, weakness	Fish, shellfish, walnuts, some vegetable oils, seeds, green leafy vegetables	n/a
Lineolic acid	Hormone synthesis, hair and skin growth	Low energy, weakness	Fish, shellfish, walnuts, vegetable oils, seeds, green leafy vegetables	n/a
Essential amino acids[3]				
Isoleucine	Muscle maintenance, blood sugar maintenance, hemoglobin synthesis	Dizziness, fatigue, irritability, headache	Meat, fish, cheese, nuts, eggs, soy	700 mg
Leucine	Hemoglobin synthesis, blood-sugar maintenance, healing	Dizziness, fatigue, irritability, headache	Corn, dairy, eggs, fish, legumes, meat, nuts, seafood, seeds, soy, whole grains	980 mg

Nutrient	Function(s)	Deficiency Symptoms	Food Sources	RDA'
Lysine	Protein synthesis, calcium absorption, bone maintenance, collagen formation	Dizziness, fatigue, appetite loss, nausea, bloodshot eyes	Meat, cheese, cod, sardines, nuts, eggs, soy	840 mg
Methionine	Protein and epinephrine synthesis	Apathy, muscle and fat loss, lethargy, edema, skin lesions, weakness	Meat, fish, dairy, whole grains	910 mg
Tryptophan	Neurotransmitter and niacin synthesis	Depression, insomnia, schizophrenia	Chocolate, oats, bananas, dried dates, dairy, meat (especially turkey), fish, peanuts	245 mg

Nutrient	Function(s)	Deficiency Symptoms	Food Sources	RDA[1]
Vitamins[2,4]				
Vitamin B_1 (thiamine)	Energy production, nerve health, DNA/RNA formation	Appetite loss, poor digestion, insomnia, chronic constipation, weight loss, depression	Fortified breads, cereals, pasta, whole grains, lean meats, fish, legumes, soy	~1 mg
Vitamin B_2, G (riboflavin)	Energy production, hemoglobin synthesis, niacin synthesis	Bloodshot eyes, skin lesions, photosensitivity	Organ meats, dairy, yeast, oily fish, eggs, dark green leafy vegetables	~1.5 mg
Vitamin B_3 (niacin)	Energy production, cellular health, blood-sugar stabilization, fatty-acid synthesis, antioxidant, detoxification, stomach-acid synthesis	Pellagra (mouth sores, skin rashes, diarrhea, and dementia)	Dairy, corn flour, dates, eggs, fish, peanuts, pork, potatoes, tomatoes, beef liver and kidney, veal, sunflower seeds	~15 mg

Nutrient	Function(s)	Deficiency Symptoms	Food Sources	RDA[1]
Vitamin B_5 (pantothenic acid)	Energy production, cholesterol synthesis, aids stress response, fatty-acid synthesis, hemoglobin synthesis	Depression, personality changes, fatigue, heart problems	Wheat germ, cheese, corn, eggs, liver, meats, peanuts, peas, soybeans	~5.5 mg
Vitamin B_7 or H (biotin)	Fatty-acid synthesis, maintenance of sweat glands, bone marrow, male gonads, blood cells, nervous tissue, hair, and skin; energy production	Fatigue, hair loss, depression, anemia, nausea, muscle pains	Organ meats, oatmeal, egg yolks, mushrooms, bananas, peanuts, soy	300 mcg

Nutrient	Function(s)	Deficiency Symptoms	Food Sources	RDA'
Vitamin B$_{12}$ (cobalamin)	Nerve-cell maintenance, amino-acid synthesis, DNA synthesis, platelet and blood-cell synthesis, folate activation	Fatigue, appetite and digestive issues, weight loss, weakness, nausea	Liver, tuna, cottage cheese, yogurt, eggs	6 mcg
Vitamin C (ascorbic acid)	Antioxidant, tissue growth and maintenance, heart maintenance, aids immune response, collagen synthesis, cholesterol moderation, folate activation, iron regulation	Tiredness, weakness, joint and muscle aches, rash on legs, bleeding gums (scurvy)	Green peppers, citrus fruits, strawberries, tomatoes, broccoli, leafy greens, potatoes	75–125 mg

Nutrient	Function(s)	Deficiency Symptoms	Food Sources	RDA[1]
Minerals[3,4]				
Calcium[5]	Bone and tooth maintenance, heartbeat maintenance, blood clotting, nerve function, muscle function, enzyme activation	Osteoporosis, muscle cramps, lethargy, poor appetite, confusion	Dairy, seaweeds, nuts, beans	> 200 mg
Cobalt	Nerve-cell maintenance, DNA synthesis, platelet and blood-cell synthesis	Fatigue, appetite and digestive issues, weight loss, weakness, nausea	Liver, tuna, cottage cheese, yogurt, eggs	Trace

Nutrient	Function(s)	Deficiency Symptoms	Food Sources	RDA'
Copper	Nerve function, energy production, elastin formation, enzyme function, blood-sugar regulation, hemoglobin synthesis, iron absorption, antioxidant	Anemia, dilated veins, low body temperature, irregular heartbeat, high cholesterol	Organ meats, seafood, beans, nuts, whole grains	1000 mcg 1.5–3 mg
Iodine	Thyroid regulation, cellular-energy usage, metabolic-rate regulation	Hypothyroidism, lethargy, weight gain	Iodized salt, shellfish, kelp	~150 mcg
Iron	Hemoglobin synthesis, oxygen transport, cellular oxidation, protein and enzyme synthesis	Fatigue, irritability, decreased immune response	Meat, salmon, beans, whole grains	~15 mg

Nutrient	Function(s)	Deficiency Symptoms	Food Sources	RDA'
Magnesium	Formation of teeth and bones, protein synthesis, energy regulation, nerve maintenance, muscle maintenance, bone maintenance	Anxiety, irritability, diarrhea, muscle spasms, abnormal heart rhythm, confusion	Soy, legumes, whole grains, green leafy vegetables, wheat bran, nuts	~300 mg
Manganese	Enzyme synthesis, protein and fat metabolism, blood-sugar regulation, immune-system support	High cholesterol, slow hair and nail growth, weight loss, dermatitis	Nuts, seeds, wheat germ, whole grains, legumes, pineapples	Trace
Phosphorus	Formation of bones and teeth, kidney and heart function, bone healing, energy regulation	Pain, joint stiffness, fatigue, numbness, irritability, weakness	Legumes, nuts, meat, poultry	~700 mg

Nutrient	Function(s)	Deficiency Symptoms	Food Sources	RDA¹
Potassium	Muscle maintenance, water balance, nerve maintenance, basic metabolism function	Weakness, nausea, irregular heartbeat, vomiting, mood swings	Fresh fish, broccoli, legumes, apples, tomatoes, potatoes, green leafy vegetables, bananas, apricots	> 780 mg
Selenium	White-blood-cell synthesis and maintenance, thyroid function, immune-system function, coreacts with vitamin E as an antioxidant	Heart disease, cataracts, premature aging	Fish, shellfish, red meat, grains, eggs, chicken, liver, garlic	70 mcg

Nutrient	Function(s)	Deficiency Symptoms	Food Sources	RDA¹
Sodium	Blood and body-fluid regulation, acid-base balance, nerve transmission, heart-activity regulation	Muscle cramps, fatigue, hair loss	Salt, meats, fish, nuts	< 500 mg

Sadly, you can't always get everything you need from your diet, so it's a good idea to take supplements that include all the vitamins, minerals, amino acids, and fatty acids you need. A well-balanced diet will usually provide all the essential nutrients your body can't synthesize, but there are occasional exceptions: consider the friend I mentioned at the beginning of this chapter who suffered from an iron deficiency. Therefore, it won't hurt to take a good multivitamin on a daily basis. If nothing else, it'll help rev up your metabolism, and can tide you over if something's deficient in your diet.

▲ ▲ ▲
▼ ▼ ▼

▼ ENERGY BANDIT #2 | A big sweet tooth

Sugar from foods such as orange juice and candy can activate your appetite instead of control it. You're getting a burst of pure sugar, which stimulates an immediate release of insulin, causing your blood sugar to drop. Soon you will feel irritable and driven to eat again.

▲ ENERGY BOOSTER | Try metabolism-boosting substitutes for your favorite foods

Try an egg-white omelet and whole-wheat toast with jam in the morning instead of sugary cereal. In the afternoon, try hard-boiled eggs, low-fat yogurt or cheese, or a protein shake. Even something as small as a few crackers can help you keep going. Here's a little ditty my mom taught me as a young girl that I have always remembered: "Fruit is sugar, rice is starch, stay away from them after dark." If you just can't seem to keep your hands out of the cookie jar:

If you like ...	Try ...
breakfast cereal	oatmeal
chips and dip	soy chips and hummus
pretzels	edamame
butter	Smart Balance Omega PLUS spread
chips	pickles (for salt) or flavored rice cakes (for crunch)
ice cream	frozen low-fat pudding cups
cake, pie	angel food cake with fruit
Popsicles	frozen fruit, such as pineapple or strawberry
using oil in baked goods	substituting applesauce

▲ ▲ ▲
▼ ▼ ▼

▼ ENERGY BANDIT #3 | Dehydration

While technically water is not a nutrient, we do not get all the water our bodies need from the food we eat, so supplementation is essential. If you feel like you're drained dry, perhaps you are. Potential symptoms of dehydration are as follows:[6]

1. Dry, sticky mouth and eyes
2. Drastically decreased urine output
3. Concentrated urine that is dark yellow
4. Blood in the stool
5. Sunken eyes
6. Severe lethargy
7. Dizziness and light-headedness
8. Confusion
9. Rapid heartbeat
10. Dry skin with markedly decreased elasticity

The last half of the list is typical of severe cases; if you have symptoms 6 through 10, seek medical help right away.

▲ ENERGY BOOSTER | **Stay hydrated**

Water is one of the most important substances that your body uses. It serves the following purposes:

- Eliminates headaches, increases energy, and decreases blood pressure. A hydrated body more easily transports oxygen and nutrients to the muscles.
- Flushes toxins out of the body. Studies show that drinking water may cut your risk for colon, breast, and bladder cancer.
- Makes you feel better overall and boosts mental performance. Mild dehydration can give you a headache and impair your ability to concentrate.
- Assists in elimination and prevents urinary-tract infections and kidney stones. Need I say more?

- Decreases the risk of strains, pulls, and muscle injuries. Water keeps muscles supple and joints lubricated.
- Aids digestion and helps the body absorb nutrients. Water causes blood to move nutrients into the kidneys rapidly.
- Helps with weight loss.

About 20 percent of the water your body needs to remain hydrated is absorbed from your food; the rest comes from beverages. In theory, maintaining hydration sounds simple: all you have to do is remember to drink plenty of water. In practice, it's hard to remember to get all the water you need, especially if you're busy doing other things, so it's best to track it. (*Bonus:* For a simple chart on tracking your water consumption, e-mail Water@TheProductivityPro.com.)

You need water most when you're most active. The average adult requires *at least* sixty-four ounces of water each day for optimal health. That's half a gallon. If you're more active than usual, or built on a larger scale than most, you may require even more water than that. There's a calculator at http://www.bottledwater.org/public/hydcal/input1.html to help you estimate how much water you need based on your weight and the amount of exercise you get. If you either drink too little water or lose too many fluids—for example, through sweating, speaking, or diarrhea—you can easily become dehydrated.

Fortunately, mild dehydration is easy to treat: all you have to do is replace your missing fluids. Despite all the marketing claims from sports-drink manufacturers, water works best for everyday hydration. However, if you find yourself seriously dehydrated, you'll need to drink an electrolyte solution; fortunately, these are available without a prescription at most pharmacies. Avoid sports drinks, because they're full of sugar, which can trigger diarrhea. Once you're rehydrated, maintenance is simple: just drink plenty of fluids every day. Coffee, tea, soft drinks, and other beverages containing caffeine or similar compounds don't count, because the caffeine can act as a diuretic, causing you to urinate more and thus dehydrate faster. Fruit juices are good in limited amounts, but don't overdo them. Like sports drinks, most commercial fruit juices are too sugary, and often contain very little real juice.

For an excellent primer on dehydration, check out http://www .nlm.nih.gov/medlineplus/ency/article/000982.htm#visualContent.

▲ ▲ ▲
▼ ▼ ▼

▼ ENERGY BANDIT #4 | An overreliance on stimulants

I'm not talking about the hard stuff here, just the everyday stimulants we surround ourselves with. The so-called energy supplements (such as Vivarin), herbal energizers, and energy drinks (such as Red Bull) sold over the counter are probably the most common ways people self-medicate low energy. The primary ingredients of all these products are caffeine, ephedrine, phenylpropanolamine, and their close relatives. If you want to maintain a steady, optimum energy level, avoid them like the plague. Your body will thank you. Other legal stimulants, like caffeinated soda, trigger a fight-or-flight reflex that releases stress hormones (epinephrine and norepinephrine) into your system. The result? A revved-up metabolism and heightened energy for a while, followed by a big energy slump.[7] Hardly worth all the trouble, especially if you take more stimulants to avoid the negative effects of earlier stimulants.

▲ ENERGY BOOSTER | Steer clear of stimulants

There's no doubt that stimulants perk you up, but they do it in a way that you have to pay for later. Most people don't realize it, but almost all of our everyday stimulants are classified as sympathomimetic

amines—a form of speed.[8] The worst offenders are phenylpropanolamine, ephedrine, and caffeine (which, incidentally, can't legally
be sold in combination).

All sympathomimetic amines temporarily elevate the following as
part of the fight-or-flight reflex[9]:

- Alertness
- Anxiety
- Heart rate
- Blood pressure
- Respiration rate
- Muscle tension
- Perspiration
- Urination
- Blood supply to skeletal muscles and brain
- Dilation of pupils and lung bronchioles
- Blood-sugar production

Things that get suppressed include the following:

- Saliva production
- Digestion
- Sexual function
- Blood supply to internal organs
- Sleep cycle
- Appetite
- Fatigue
- Concentration

All these physiological responses are intended to help you survive,
one way or another, in the face of a dire threat. Triggering them with
stimulants can result in exhaustion and energy drain in the short
run, and a laundry list of negative effects in the long run, including
depression, chronic fatigue syndrome, and dehydration, all of which

are energy stealers—and they're among the least of the bad effects you can expect.

▲ ▲ ▲
▼ ▼ ▼

| **Drinking too much alcohol**

You may feel calm after you've had several alcoholic drinks, but those drinks will disrupt your sleep and cause low energy the next day. Alcohol is also a depressant; it'll suppress your entire nervous system (and your energy) rather than stimulate it. In addition, it has numerous other physical effects that can drag down your energy: it can dehydrate you and destabilize your blood-sugar level, and there are indications that it can actually inhibit energy production at a cellular level. This isn't to say that you should never take a drink again; just be careful about how much you imbibe, in social situations or otherwise. For all you ever wanted to know about but were afraid to ask, visit the National Institute on Alcohol Abuse and Alcoholism at http://www.niaaa.nih.gov/.

▲ ENERGY BOOSTER | **Limit your alcohol consumption**

Will the occasional beer or glass of wine with dinner hurt you? Not really, but too much alcohol at any one time can negatively impact your energy level for a day or more. Here are a few relatively painless ways to cut down on your alcohol consumption in social situations:

- Drink out of tall, thin glasses like flutes. This works as well for cutting alcohol consumption as it does for decreasing general caloric intake (see chapter 2).
- Stick to drinks with a lower alcohol content, such as a shot mixed with soda or juice, rather than just the shot.

- Pace your drinking; that is, sip instead of chugging, so your drinks last longer.
- Drink plenty of water between alcoholic drinks. Not only will this dilute the alcohol, it will help you avoid the worst effects of alcohol-derived dehydration.
- Eat something as you drink—but avoid those bar nuts. They're intended to make you drink more, to counteract their saltiness.
- Instead of a glass of wine, have a red wine spritzer (five ounces of red wine mixed with club soda).

▼ ENERGY BANDIT #6 | **Smoking**

Smoking is arguably the nastiest of the legal addictions, in many different ways. Sure, nicotine delivers a quick burst of energy, but it's hardly worth the price your body has to pay. In the long term, smoking causes diseases and conditions that limit a person's ability to be active—or worse. Consider, for example, the wholesale damage that occurs to a smoker's lungs, resulting in a wide range of ailments from emphysema to cancer. Aside from all the other health effects, these diseases can limit your ability to absorb oxygen, which is essential to breaking down food and nutrients. Smoking also introduces carbon monoxide (CO) into the bloodstream, and CO is far more efficient at binding to the hemoglobin in red blood cells than oxygen is. Since one of hemoglobin's major tasks is the delivery of oxygen to your cells, it's easy to see how too much CO in the bloodstream can generate lower levels of energy body-wide.

▲ ENERGY BOOSTER | **Stop smoking!**

While there are undeniable physiological addictions associated with smoking, keep in mind that it's called a "habit" for good reason. Part of the reason you smoke (assuming you do) is that you're used to doing it; that being the case, there are many, many things you can do to occupy your time and hands instead of smoking. Just make sure you don't turn to another energy-destroying habit. Instead, try some of these activities when the urge to smoke strikes:

- Eat a celery stalk, or some other low-calorie food.
- Chew on a toothpick.
- Chew some sugarless gum.
- Eat some sunflower seeds.
- Call a friend.
- Go for a walk.
- Take a shower.
- Do a crossword puzzle.
- Chug some ice water.
- Remind yourself why you need to stop.

It's all replacement therapy, but it helps. You'll find a list of 101 things to do instead of smoking at http://quitsmoking.about.com/od/cravingsandurges/a/101thingstodo.htm.

Alternatively, you can start your own program. Write down your current activity level (e.g., two packs of cigarettes per day). Then determine your twenty-one-day goal at the end of this program (e.g., ten cigarettes per day), your three-month goal (one pack per week), and your one-year goal (quit). Last, decide what wonderful rewards you will give yourself for your efforts. Use the money you previously spent on the addiction for something you've wanted for a long time: a new kitchen counter, a dining room table, a landscaped yard, and so forth. Do something fun with the extra time you will have: go dancing, take yoga classes, try karate, catch up on a former hobby you've put aside.

While smoking is probably one of the hardest addictions to break, it's crucial to stop, so you can start feeling good again. If you can succeed in at least cutting back, you'll soon see an increase in your physical energy. For the whole story on smoking, visit http://health.nih.gov/result.asp/605.

▲ ▲ ▲
▼ ▼ ▼

▼ ENERGY BANDIT #7 | Making it inconvenient to eat nutritiously

If you're working hard to increase your energy level through good nutritional habits, make it easier to succeed. Start by limiting the worst energy stealers in your environment.

▲ ENERGY BOOSTER | Focus on convenience

- If you hate making salad but want to eat it for its nutritional value, buy prewashed greens and always have a bag on hand. That way you don't have the excuse that it's too much of a hassle.
- Set yourself up to eat nutritiously. Wash, cut, and bag up veggies and fruits each week. If you buy a cantaloupe at the store but pass it up at home in favor of Froot Loops, make it easier on yourself to make good choices by having serving sizes already prepared in individual Baggies you can quickly grab before you change your mind.
- Grab and go. I like those premade light tuna salad kits. More expensive, yes, but worth it—I can't make excuses about how

much hassle it is to prepare, and it's much more nutritious than grabbing a candy bar from the vending machine.

▲ ▲ ▲
▼ ▼ ▼

Surrounding yourself with temptations

The trickiest part of eating high-energy, metabolism-boosting foods is my children—not that my eating is their fault, but the treats they like are tempting. I try to be a good role model for healthy eating, but I also don't want to deprive them of the occasional treats other children enjoy. The downside is if there's junk food all around me, I'm more likely to eat it.

Clear your house of junk

My mother-in-law will buy a box of treats, eat one or two, and then bring the rest over to our house "for the children." Or she will make lots of holiday goodies and tell me to freeze them. So we give a few to the children and toss the rest in the trash. Mom feels good for having brought them over, and we feel good that we didn't eat them. It's important to create an environment that's conducive to nutrition:

- Keep sugary and high-fat snacks out of your cupboard. If junk food isn't easily accessible, you're less likely to eat it and more likely to eat food with higher nutritional value.
- The same goes for when you're at work: if you get hungry and don't have anything to eat, you are bound to end up in front of the vending machine or in your car in the fast-food

lane. Stock up on a stash of healthy food you can keep in your desk drawer for just such an emergency: almonds; raisins; fiber cereal; tuna packets in water; fruit cups in water; dried fruit; power bars; whole fruit; and raw, ready-to-go vegetables like carrots, celery, sweet bell peppers, and tomatoes.

- Clear out your liquor cabinet.
- Get rid of the beer in the fridge.
- Throw out the cigarettes.
- Don't let caffeinated beverages into your house.
- Avoid all stimulants, including diet pills.
- If you're hooked on soda, try water flavored with lemon or lime or seltzer water.

▲ ▲ ▲

Four

Exercise

Physiology quiz item #4:
I'm too tired to exercise

It will infuse your energy and boost your mood. It will help you lose weight and decrease your risk of disease. It's a miracle! But 80 percent of Americans don't take it, even at its lowest dosage. It's exercise. I know, I know—you're tired of hearing about how important exercise is for your energy level, but you're going to hear it again. If you're consistently low on energy, an ironic paradox is that the less active you are, the less energy you will have. A sedentary lifestyle contributes greatly to fatigue. According to the Centers for Disease Control and Prevention, more than 50 percent of American adults do not get the recommended amount of physical activity a day and 25 percent of Americans aren't physically active at all.[1] A study from the VU Medical Center in Amsterdam of 1,747 full-time workers showed that strenuous leisure-time physical activity might play a role in the prevention of future psychological complaints, poor general health, and long-term absenteeism in a working population.[2]

If you are feeling exhausted, getting some exercise will give you the energy you need. Exercise speeds up blood flow and your breathing rate, which in turn brings more oxygen to your heart, lungs, brain, and muscles. Oxygen is your friend. It perks you up—more energy. Regular aerobic activity—such as running, walking, tennis, biking, gardening, or sports—will make you more alert. Figure out how to move. And move daily.

▼ ▼ ▼

▼ ENERGY BANDIT #1 | **Lack of regular aerobic activity**

Doing aerobics (or cardiovascular activity) involves large movements of your arms, legs, and hips. Your aerobic fitness level refers to the ability of your heart, blood vessels, and lungs (cardiovascular system) to supply fuel during sustained physical activity.

▲ ENERGY BOOSTER | **Do *something* for thirty minutes**

According to the Mayo Clinic, aerobic exercise strengthens your heart and lungs and improves blood flow. Regular aerobic exercise also releases endorphins, which are your body's natural painkillers. People who exercise regularly are less susceptible to minor viral illnesses, such as colds and flu. If you feel down or depressed, aerobic exercise will boost your mood and reduce the tension you feel. Exercise can increase your stamina, reduce fatigue, and help you relax.[3] Better yet, a November 2006 study in the *Journal of Gerontology: Medical Sciences* reported that people who get as little as three hours of aerobic activity each week have a better memory, are better at switching between mental tasks, and can screen out distractions better than people who do not exercise.[4] During cardiovascular exercise, the locus coeruleus in your brain keeps you going by kicking up production of norepinephrine, a chemical that makes you feel alert and energetic.

For years, the medical community has preached the need for vigorous aerobic activity and athletic fitness, with many experts requiring six or more hours per week. Perhaps that's why you don't work out now—it feels too self-defeating. Good news! Numerous studies now show that you don't always have to break a sweat to reap the most significant health benefits of exercise. With very little effort—around thirty minutes a day—you can make a dramatic improvement in your health and energy level. The biggest health benefits come from a small increase in energy level. How much of an increase? According to a study reported in the *Journal of Medical Science and Exercise,* most of the benefits of exercise kick in with the first 1,000 calories of increased activity each week, which reduces your risk of dying by 20 to 30 percent.[5] So, how do you burn an extra 1,000 calories per week? That's easy! It equates to 145 calories per day, an easy number to hit just by doing regular activities. There are great exercise calculators at www.caloriesperhour.com and www.caloriecontrol.org/exercalc.html, where you choose an activity, enter how long you're going to do it and your weight, and voilà! The trick is to make sure you're doing *something* every day, or double the requirement to 300 calories every other day.

If thirty minutes of daily activity is too daunting, break it into two fifteen-minute or three ten-minute sessions. How about doing one fifteen-minute session before work and one fifteen-minute session after work? In experiments conducted by Robert Thayer, Ph.D., at California State University, and reported in his book *Calm Energy: How People Regulate Mood with Food and Exercise* (Oxford University Press, 2003), a brisk ten-minute walk not only increased energy, but the effects lasted up to two hours. And when the daily ten-minute walks continued for three weeks, overall energy levels and mood were lifted.

Bottom line: Do what you love! What did you like to do as a child? Ride a bike? Roller skate? Play tag? Jump on a trampoline? Walk? Run? Maybe you enjoy exercise classes? Yoga? Pilates? Shooting hoops? Toning? Swimming? Anything that forces you to move around is beneficial. Try a lot of different activities until you find the right mix of exercise for you. Enjoyment is the key to long-term commitment.

▲ ▲ ▲

▼ ▼ ▼

▼ ENERGY BANDIT #2 | ## Relying on your car to get you everywhere

Get out of the habit of jumping into your car to drive down the street or around the block. Stop driving and start walking.

▲ ENERGY BOOSTER | ## Buy a pedometer

This is a fun way to check how much you're moving every day. Most people average between 2,000 and 3,000 steps per day. You want to move at least 6,000 steps per day, and 10,000 steps per day if you're trying to lose weight. Wear your pedometer all the time and glance down at it to see how you're doing. Keep a log and challenge yourself toward a particular goal each day. Find little ways to add more steps to your counter, like taking the stairs instead of the elevator and walking the dog instead of letting it out. You'll be amazed at how quickly those steps add up. Here are some other creative ways to get moving:

- Walk during your lunch break.
- Force yourself to park far away from the entrance to the mall or grocery store (instead of driving around in circles for five minutes trying to find the closest spot).
- Watch TV from your treadmill (my husband's favorite trick).
- Walk around the block to get the mail.
- Meet your friends for a walk.
- Walk up and down a flight of stairs for ten minutes.
- Choose the farthest entrance to your building and park in the last spot.
- When you need a copy machine or restroom, go to one on a different floor.

- Take a couple of ten-minute breaks during the day to walk a few laps around your floor.
- Walk over to see a colleague rather than send an e-mail.
- Get up and walk over to the TV to change the channel instead of using a remote.
- Walk around your office while using a speakerphone.
- Walk to any destination that is less than one mile away.
- Don't take the moving walkways at the airport.
- Take the kids out for a family walk after dinner.
- Unload groceries from the car in several trips.
- Talk to your friend on a cordless phone and walk around the house.
- While your kids are playing soccer, walk around the field perimeter.

▲　▲　▲
▼　▼　▼

▼ ENERGY BANDIT #3 | **You don't lift weights**

An important way to feel more energetic is to build stronger muscles through weight training. The more you pump weights, the more muscle you will build. The more muscle you have, the higher your resting metabolism. The higher your metabolism, the more energy you have throughout the day—even sitting at your desk. As one researcher puts it, a pound of lean muscle mass is metabolic gold; it takes up less space than other tissues, but requires more energy output. Fat, on the other hand, is like a pile of feathers; it is low-maintenance, but it takes up more space in your body, and doesn't contribute significantly to your physical energy budget.[6] Weak muscles can lead to fatigue and reduced energy. Strong muscles lead to bone strength and reduced risk of injury. Spending more time at our desks instead of working in physically demanding jobs has caused our muscles to become soft, weak, and tight. This sedentary lifestyle contributes greatly to fatigue. Lifting weights speeds up oxygen flow to your heart, lungs, and brain, which perks you up. Plus, it will boost flexibility and help firm your body. After working out, when your blood and oxygen are flowing to your muscles, you will feel totally "pumped up"!

▲ ENERGY BOOSTER | **Include weights in your fitness routine**

You might feel intimidated to join a gym, where your first tour made it obvious that *everyone* knew how to use all those complex-looking machines. You didn't want to look ridiculous, so you didn't join. Too bad you didn't know that most gyms provide a complimentary session with a fitness instructor, who would show you how to use everything. If not, you can sign up for a personal-training session, and within an hour you'll be working out on the machines with the best of them. Should you use the free weights? If you're a beginner, you might want to start with the fixed machines. You can add free weights as you get more familiar with the exercises and want to work specific muscles.

Many people work an entire circuit for their entire body all at once. The gym *Curves* uses this concept. Others rotate the lower and upper body, alternating every other day. A good beginning work-out could include the following:

- Chest (bench press)
- Shoulders (seated dumbbell press)
- Back (dumbbell rows)
- Triceps (seated dumbbell extensions)
- Glutes (squats)
- Biceps (seated dumbbell curls)
- Thighs (leg presses)
- Hamstrings (leg curls)
- Calves (leg lifts)

▲ ▲ ▲

▼ ▼ ▼

▼ ENERGY BANDIT #4 | You don't make time for fitness

You hear yourself saying "I'm too busy" or "I don't have enough time." Everything else in your life seems to crowd out this essential energy activity.

▲ ENERGY BOOSTER | Sneak in fitness

While reading an article in a magazine or newspaper, I stand up and do squats. It really tones my thighs and doesn't take any time away from the activity I would have been doing anyway. Squeeze in little fitness opportunities throughout the day today:

- When you arrive home from the grocery store, do a few biceps curls with each full plastic bag before you set it down.
- If you need to go to the restroom, don't use the closest bathroom—use the one that requires you to walk a bit, preferably up the stairs.
- Balance on one foot the entire length of time (two minutes, hopefully) you're brushing your teeth. Then stand on the other foot while you brush your hair. This is great for core stabilization.
- Invest in a cordless headset. When I get a call, I can chat while walking around my house and doing lunges.
- Install a chin-up bar in a doorway in your home. Every time you pass it by, do as many chin-ups as you can (even if it's none to start—you'll get there).
- While talking on the phone, do knee bends or squats until you hang up (this might force you to reduce the length of the call).
- Go to a sporting-goods store and buy two inexpensive light-

weight dumbbells. Every time you feel stiff, take a break and do a quick set of ten overhead presses. The tension will fade away and your energy will return.

Most people complain about not having enough time because they are thinking about trying to find a "block of time" in which to exercise. You'll rarely have a sixty-minute block magically appear on your calendar. How about ten minutes? Surely you can find ten minutes a few times a day to move around a bit. Do *something*! If you can't find ten minutes, you're making up excuses. You say you want to increase your energy? Put your time where your mouth is!

▼ ENERGY BANDIT #5 | You're in a workout rut

"Exercise is so boring." Sound familiar? Boredom was once my biggest fitness challenge and my greatest rationalization to not do it. My only exercise was walking on the treadmill in the living room while watching the *Today* show in the morning. I got tired of the same old thing and stopped doing it. It's also quite easy for me to make excuses about not working out while I'm on the road: I'm too tired; I've worked hard all day; I deserve to veg out in front of a movie and eat pie in my room instead of exercising; there is no gym in this hotel. All of which results in stagnant energy on the road.

▲ ENERGY BOOSTER | Change it up a bit

Maybe your body has become used to the same level of effort through the same old exercise routine. Doing the same fitness routine week after week isn't only boring; it can lead to a training plateau in which your body eventually becomes acclimated to the exercises, so you see fewer gains. So change it up a bit. I had been going to the gym at my city's recreation center (the membership is included in my association dues). It was always the same old thing, the same old scenery, the same old machines. So I signed up for an adult ballet class at my recreation center on Thursday evenings. I also joined a Lady Fitness gym just five minutes from my home and found a Saturday-morning yoga class I love. The key is to do something different! Hit the up arrow on the treadmill. Alternate your walk with some backward walking and skipping. Toss another weight on the machine. Alternate bike rides with jogging. Go to the pool now and then. Change your walking course: go in a different direction or on a totally different route. I also use an Xbox 360 program called "Yourself Fitness" and work out with my virtual personal trainer, Maya. My husband, John, is an avid weight lifter, so I started showing him weight routines from my *Shape* magazine subscription. He agreed to help me do the programs a couple of times a week. Now I'm having fun working out, doing a *lot* of different activities, and looking forward to the next event.

▲ ▲ ▲
▼ ▼ ▼

▼ ENERGY BANDIT #6 | You don't exercise when you travel

"I travel too much and am in unfamiliar places." My speaking colleague, Janelle Barlow, a branding expert, makes exercise a major commitment while she travels and figures out a way to make it happen. She's a swimmer, so she shops in advance for hotels with good swimming pools. She asks lots of questions before making a decision, such as operating hours, length, temperature, and so forth. She will go out of her way or stay farther away from the client site just to have a good pool. Some pools even have adults-only hours, like my favorite Embassy Suites in San Antonio, Texas.

▲ ENERGY BOOSTER | Create a travel workout plan

If I work out while on the road, I feel rejuvenated and more equipped to tackle the day. My travel aches and pains and muscle tightness and lethargy all seem to vanish. I gain less weight, sleep more soundly, and have more strength for schlepping my luggage across the airport. My husband, John, absolutely cannot travel without working out or his stress level will skyrocket, making him no fun to vacation with. The trick is to make it easy, assume you're going to do it, and plan accordingly. Here are some considerations:

- Where should you stay, the Marriott, Hilton, or Day's Inn? Book your hotel based on the availability of workout rooms and pools. The hotel chains that report that they have *on-site* workout facilities at ALL of their properties are the Crowne Plaza, Four Seasons, Hilton, Homewood Suites, Red Lion, Ritz-Carlton, Sheraton, Summerfield Suites, and Wingate.[7] Some hotels also have partnerships with nearby workout facilities to offer day passes as part of your hotel stay.

- What should you pack? If you don't have a choice of where to stay, and your hotel doesn't have a workout facility, not to worry. Pack a jump rope, a rubber exercise tube, and a pair of water-filled dumbbells (emptied, of course). You can jump rope, lift, and stretch. Make the most of where you are by running on the beach, taking a walking tour of the city, or climbing the hotel stairs instead of using the elevator. Worst case, you can do sit-ups, push-ups, jumping jacks, and other old-fashioned calisthenics from your PE days in high school. To avoid the excuse that workout gear is clunky, buy a pair of tennis shoes that fold flat. Look for the new "minimalist" type of shoes that don't have the same rigid qualities as older-model tennis shoes. If the facility has a pool, the only workout gear you'll need is your swimsuit.

- How can I make room for it in my schedule? Plan your flights carefully. I always schedule my plane to arrive in the early evening, so that by the time I get my bags, go to the hotel, and get settled, it's time for a decent bedtime. Then I've had enough sleep to hit the gym before my work commitments. I'll often read some work items while walking on the treadmill. Make sure to drink plenty of water on the flight, where the humidity is less than 10 percent, so that you're not dehydrated and exhausted at the end of your trip.

▲ ▲ ▲
▼ ▼ ▼

▼ ENERGY BANDIT #7 | Lack of discipline

My husband, John, likes to exercise in the morning because, he says, if he doesn't do it then, it doesn't happen. However, John doesn't like to get out of bed in the morning! When the alarm clock goes off at 6:30 AM, he's content to turn it off and roll over for more shuteye. However, if he knows he has his workout partner waiting for him, he will get up every time (sometimes accompanied by a lot of groaning), so as not to disappoint his friend. Once his workout partner went on an extended business trip to Germany for several weeks . . . guess how many times John worked out. It was somewhere less than twice. Without a workout partner, his discipline isn't strong.

▲ ENERGY BOOSTER | Get a workout buddy

There really is power in working out with other people: a friend, a family member, or a personal trainer. Even a virtual one, like my personal trainer, Maya. Another reason I like working out with Maya is that she's tough. After each Thursday workout, for example, she'll say, "See you Friday." And if I don't log in on Friday, she scolds me!

Better yet, when I do as she asks, I get "rewards" like better music choices and new environments to work out in. I remember wanting to work out with the "Hawaiian Paradise" background. She made me complete ten scheduled workouts before the game unlocked that level as a reward. So ask a friend if he or she wants to be your lifting or walking partner, and see how much more disciplined you will become. Some health clubs offer a matchmaking service of sorts, pairing members for regular workouts. In addition to having someone to talk with, the time will go more quickly. Having a workout buddy will also increase your discipline, knowing there is someone waiting for you. Research has shown that people trying to lose weight are likelier to stick with diet and exercise if they buddy up with someone who has already successfully lost weight. Better yet, pay a personal trainer to meet you at the gym. You're more likely to show up if you've already forked out the bucks!

▼ ENERGY BANDIT #8 | You're just not motivated to work out

Perhaps you're feeling lazy. Perhaps it hurts. Maybe you just don't like it. For whatever reason, there are occasions when you just don't feel like exercising. Getting yourself off the couch might require an incentive.

▲ ENERGY BOOSTER | Give yourself a reward

Play silly games with yourself. For example, allow yourself to listen to your iPod only when you're working out. If I want to watch television, I require myself to be walking on my treadmill in front of it the entire time it's on. Perhaps you could get an audio book of a novel you want to read but allow yourself to listen to it only when you're on your treadmill or running. Promise yourself a massage if you meet your goal of hitting the gym three times a week for a month. Buy yourself that new outfit you want if you lose five pounds. Treat yourself to a round of golf with your buddies if you stick to your food plan this week. Tape your favorite show and allow yourself to watch it only while working out. You get the picture: anything you find tantalizing should do the trick and aid your discipline.

▲ ▲ ▲

Five

Metabolism

Physiology quiz item #5:
I keep going and going and going

Just like an Eveready battery, you want to keep going and going and going all day long. To achieve that goal, however, you need to super-charge your metabolism and keep it revving in high gear. This process isn't necessarily easy, and it requires an understanding of your own biochemical makeup and metabolism.

In its simplest sense, the term *metabolism* describes the cellular processes that convert the calories in the food you eat into energy you need to get through the day. When you're sitting on the couch watching television, your metabolism is idling. When you're running uphill, it's in overdrive. Your resting metabolism is the energy it takes to simply sustain your basic bodily functions. It accounts for 60 to 75 percent of your total daily calorie burn and depends on several factors, such as body weight, diet, gender, and age. Another 15 to 30 percent of your daily calorie burn is governed by your activity level and exercise. And 10 percent of your daily burn goes to digesting your food.

The rate of metabolism varies from person to person—among other things, gender, age, amount of muscle mass, and how much you exercise will all affect your metabolic rate, but that doesn't mean you can't tweak it for maximal performance.

▼ ▼ ▼

Not knowing how to boost your metabolism

Human metabolism can be broken down into three basic subcategories:

- Thermal effect of food (TEF), the energy used to process our meals
- Resting metabolic rate (RMR), which includes the calories used to maintain all our tissues and autonomic processes
- Physical activity energy expenditure (PAEE), the calories we use to provide energy for physical activity[1]

There's not much you can do to change your TEF, but RMR and PAEE can be manipulated. Your metabolic rate is regulated by more than just your calorie intake, but just how the various factors will affect you can be hard to pin down. Changing your diet without changing other aspects of your lifestyle won't necessarily result in a higher metabolic rate; if you trigger the wrong hormonal changes and muscle loss, you'll end up with a lower metabolic rate than you started out with—and correspondingly less energy.

▲ ENERGY BOOSTER | **Practice the power of eight**

If you want to increase your endurance and stamina and stay alert longer, practice these tips on a daily basis:

- Exercise vigorously, which will increase your cardiovascular activity and help you burn fat.
- Lift weights to build energy-producing lean muscle mass.

- Eat five or six small meals a day. Don't skip meals, especially breakfast.
- Make sure your meals have a healthy mix of high-energy proteins and carbohydrates, with a little bit of fat to slow digestion and give a feeling of satiety.
- Drink your minimum daily requirement of water.
- Eliminate stimulants.
- Cut back on caffeinated drinks, especially coffee and soda. Decaffeinated herbal tea is fine, especially green tea.

You've seen most of these tips before in other chapters, but they bear repeating. Following them won't necessarily result in an immediate increase in your energy endurance, but after a few days you *will* start to notice a difference. As with everything else you do, you'll need to work on increasing your metabolism a bit at a time.

▲ ▲ ▲
▼ ▼ ▼

▼ ENERGY BANDIT #2 | Too little blood glucose

Your energy level is governed by one key component of your metabolism: your blood-sugar level (a.k.a. blood-glucose level). This is a measure of the amount of glucose in your bloodstream, and is most often rendered in milligrams per deciliter of blood (mg/dL). As your body's primary chemical fuel, glucose is used for everything from making your heart beat to helping you eliminate waste—but if there's too much of it in your bloodstream, it turns into a surprisingly vicious poison.

Your body functions properly within a fairly narrow blood-sugar range, like a well-tuned organic machine that performs only when the fuel mix is neither too lean nor too rich. That range is about 80–120 mg/dL. Too much sugar intake can teach your body to become less efficient at using the sugar it receives, leaving you with both less energy and the long-term effects of damage. Too little blood sugar, or an inability to transport it into your cells, can rob you of energy altogether.[2] Through a series of complicated biochemical feedback mechanisms, your body will, with rare exceptions, keep the fuel mix where it needs to be.

Not surprisingly, too little glucose in your bloodstream means you're not getting enough of the fuel your body needs, and so you can start to feel listless—and in some cases, really weird. Any blood-sugar level below 70 mg/dL is considered too low for your body to function optimally, and, depending on how low your blood sugar gets, symptoms may include the following:

- Anxiety
- Physical weakness
- Hunger
- Nervousness
- Shakiness
- Perspiration (cold sweat)
- Dizziness/light-headedness
- Sleepiness
- Confusion
- Trouble speaking

Some people suffer from a chronic lack of blood sugar, which goes by the name of hypoglycemia. Ironically, diabetics—people who suffer from a consistent *excess* of blood sugar—often have hypoglycemic episodes that are triggered when their medications scavenge glucose from their bloodstream too effectively. Clearly, hypoglycemia can be a serious problem, but the symptoms usually go away quickly once you get your blood sugar to a reasonable level. It's fairly simple to do this with a few glucose tablets, a piece of candy, or some fruit juice.

▲ ENERGY BOOSTER | **Keep a stash at your desk**

Keep energy sources on hand for those "just in case" times when you feel your blood sugar plummet. For example, cut up a power bar into "fingers" and eat one every forty-five minutes. This will keep the furnace stoked. Or have a power snack if you need to eat between scheduled meals. Choose a treat that combines protein, a little fat, and some fiber, such as tuna with light mayo on crackers, peanut butter on whole-wheat bread, or a handful of nuts with a glass of low-fat (not skim) milk. The carbs give you a quick pick-me-up, the protein keeps your energy up, and the fat makes the energy last.

Even those of us whose bodies are usually vigilant about maintaining proper blood-sugar levels can hit a low point if we miss a meal or imbibe too much alcohol without accompanying it with food. (Alcohol, which is made up almost entirely of carbohydrates, has the perverse effect of lowering blood sugar in the long run.)

▲ ▲ ▲
▼ ▼ ▼

▼ ENERGY BANDIT #3 | **Too much blood glucose**

We've all had the occasional binge on chocolate bunnies at Easter, or those scrumptious Christmas cookies Mom makes. What happens? At least temporarily, you're subject to the opposite of hypoglycemia, which is *hyper*glycemia. You'll probably be keyed up, nervous, maybe a little queasy—but those feelings will pass in an hour or two, as your body grabs that extra glucose and gets it into the cells where it's needed, or at least stores it as fat. In normal circumstances, too much glucose will give you a "sugar rush" that results in a temporary energy burst. You'll end up suffering a minor energy loss later to compensate. In some cases, however, the problem is chronic. Millions of Americans are currently living with type 2 diabetes.

▲ ENERGY BOOSTER | Get checked for diabetes

Some people have a metabolic dysfunction and simply cannot process glucose properly. This condition is known as diabetes, and it occurs when the body lacks insulin, which locks onto special receptors on each cell and lets the glucose in to do its work. Insulin is a necessary "key" that lets glucose molecules pass through cell membranes. If the key is warped or missing, it can have a devastating effect on your energy level and general health. Glucose can't get inside the cells that need it, so it builds up in the bloodstream until it becomes poisonous. This is known as glucotoxicity. If your blood sugar exceeds 250 mg/dL for more than a few minutes, the resulting glucotoxicity can damage your internal organs and nerves. If not immediately taken care of, it can be life-threatening.

Diabetes is really more a constellation of diseases than a single illness. In some cases, it sneaks up on its victim and strikes suddenly, with an unpredictable autoimmune reaction that kills all the islet cells in the pancreas. Suddenly, insulin is no longer available to open up the cells so that glucose can get inside; your blood sugar skyrockets, and you get sick. This is called type 1 diabetes. It's a point mutation, which means it's not inherited or inheritable, and it usually strikes children.

Type 2 diabetes makes itself known somewhat more slowly. Its victims usually produce plenty of insulin, but the body doesn't use the insulin properly; the little insulin keys won't open the entry locks in the cells. This is known as insulin resistance. A surprisingly large portion of the American population suffers from type 2 diabetes, which is often associated with obesity, lack of exercise, and too much intake of high-carbohydrate, low-nutrient foods.

Listed below are some symptoms of diabetes:

- Increased thirst
- Constant hunger
- Frequent urination (especially at night)

- General tiredness and fatigue
- Headaches
- Blurred vision
- Mood swings and depression
- Tingling, burning, and itching sensations in the extremities
- Slow healing
- A tendency toward skin infections
- Significant weight change, up or down, in a short period

If you feel that you may have diabetes or prediabetes, then you should run—not walk—to your doctor's office and have your blood sugar checked. A simple blood test can tell you whether or not it's out of whack.[3] Yes, the test can be a little expensive, but better a costly false alarm than to run around risking glucotoxicity. Fatigue will set in, and your liver, kidneys, eyes, nerves, and many other parts of your body might be damaged before you can react properly. Much of that damage is irreversible. Fortunately, diabetes can be controlled through the vigorous application of what doctors call the "Treatment Triad": diet, exercise, and medication.

▲ ▲ ▲
▼ ▼ ▼

▼ ENERGY BANDIT #4 | **Poor meal scheduling**

At one time or another, we've all been so busy that we've skipped a meal. Maybe you slept late and had to rush to get to school or work on time; maybe it was a simple matter of working through lunch when a difficult project monopolized your attention. Whatever the reason, when you skip a meal you end up depriving your body of the steady source of glucose—and, therefore, the energy—it needs to function properly. You wouldn't be surprised if your computer stopped working during a power outage, or your car ground to a halt when it ran out of gas, so why should you be surprised when you run out of energy as a result of not eating regularly? Like a savvy driver, you should never let your energy level touch "E" on the fuel gauge.

▲ ENERGY BOOSTER | **Stabilize your blood sugar**

The healthiest way to maintain a consistently high energy level is to keep your blood sugar steady throughout the day. Here are some suggestions to help keep you from running out of energy when you can least afford to:

- Always eat your morning meal. There's a reason why we call it "breakfast": you're breaking your overnight fast. Your waking blood-sugar level will be the lowest it's going to be all day—unless, of course, you skip breakfast and let it drop farther. People who eat breakfast are not only more energetic, they're better able to control their food intake later in the day—which means they gain less weight.[4] Needless to say, excess weight can be a significant energy stealer, even if you're not obese. If you don't eat breakfast, your hunger will increase over the course of the morning, resulting in powerful cravings at lunch that cause you to demolish the entire bowl of bar nuts and finish off the bread basket during your meeting. Mireille Guiliano asserts in her book *French Women Don't Get Fat* that because they eat balanced meals throughout the day and don't snack, French women keep their metabolism sure and steady.
- Don't skip *any* meals; this interrupts the steady flow of glucose, which can be a recipe for disaster. And eat meals at the same times every day, when possible. The body thrives on schedules and consistency.
- Instead of aiming for three big meals, go for five or six smaller ones. Snacks count, as long as they're healthy. This will cut back on the urge to binge, and help you maintain a

proper diet. Five or six small meals spaced out about every three hours should be your target. For more clues about maintaining a proper diet, see chapter 2.

While it may not always be possible to maintain a consistently high energy level all day long, these habits can help you smooth out the peaks and valleys in your metabolism. Well-balanced meals, regularly scheduled, will do wonders to make you feel more energetic during the day. Of course, you'll need to combine this tactic with other sensible options in order to get the best effect.

▲ ▲ ▲
▼ ▼ ▼

▼ ENERGY BANDIT #5 | Too many "sleepy" foods in your diet

Foods such as pasta, toast, bagels, cookies, muffins, and honey buns all qualify as sleepy foods, because they contain high levels of refined flour and sugar. When you eat them, you'll likely end up short of the fuel you need to function consistently well. Your body quickly and easily digests the carbohydrates in these products, dumping a huge amount of glucose into your bloodstream. For a while you feel jazzed up and energized; then, an hour later, you crash and burn. So what the heck happened? You've introduced too much glucose into your body all at once. Your automatic protective systems go into action to protect your body from glucotoxicity, sucking the sugar out of your bloodstream and into the muscles and liver. In its zeal to clean up the sugary excess, your body overshoots: it sucks away too much glucose, resulting in a net loss, and you experience a blood-sugar crash.

▲ ENERGY BOOSTER | Eat high-energy foods

Limit your simple carbohydrates while increasing your high-energy foods. High-energy foods are better than their low-energy counterparts, for the simple reason that they load the nutrients and fuel that you need into smaller packages. The result? Quicker energy with less waste. Go to the grocery store and fill your cart with these high-energy food choices:

- *Meat.* There's no better source of protein. Your resting metabolic rate (RMR) increases two to three times more after eating protein than it does after eating carbohydrates and fat. If you're a vegetarian, see your doctor for appropriate meat-free alternatives.
- *Concord grapes.* They enhance memory and problem-solving skills by increasing dopamine in the brain. They're also high in protective antioxidants.
- *Soy milk.* It speeds your learning ability and boosts memory (only in women, as it contains phytoestrogen).
- *Raisins.* They contain boron, which may sharpen memory and increase mental alertness and reaction time.
- *Spinach.* It's loaded with lutein and other antioxidants that protect brain cells.
- *Blueberries.* They may increase brain-cell production in the hippocampus, the area of the brain that regulates memory.
- *Bananas.* They're a good source of potassium and vitamin B_6, which helps replenish oxygen-rich red blood cells.
- *Broccoli, red and yellow peppers, and tomatoes.* All these veggies are chock-full of phytochemicals and antioxidants, which are crucial for energy production.

▲ ▲ ▲

▼ ▼ ▼

▼ ENERGY BANDIT #6 | A ho-hum metabolism

Sometimes your metabolism is just sluggish and needs a little boost.

▲ ENERGY BOOSTER | Eat spicy foods and drink green tea

Few food items can increase the human metabolic rate on their own, but two that are proven to do so are spicy foods and green tea. Of the two, green tea is by far superior. Spicy foods do temporarily boost the metabolism a bit, but they seem to play a more significant role in making healthy food more palatable. Green tea, on the other hand, has a more direct effect on the metabolism, bumping it up enough to burn a noticeable number of calories per day. Because the effect is slight—four to five cups of green tea may burn an extra sixty calories or so—it's best to take green tea extract, so you can get more bang for your buck. Some researchers say drinking two cups of green tea a day will reduce your Alzheimer's risk by 50 percent. Green tea extract can be purchased at most health-food stores for a moderate price. For more information on the green tea resolution, check out this site: http://thyroid.about.com/cs/dietweightloss/a/greentea.htm.

▲ ▲ ▲
▼ ▼ ▼

▼ ENERGY BANDIT #7 | Your afternoon trip to Starbucks

I'm at a bit of a disadvantage here, since I *love* coffee. Besides that, it's really hard to figure out what to say, since different research studies say different things about the drug. (Did I say drug? Okay, maybe a recreational chemical?) Caffeine has been shown to boost energy, improve performance on tasks, raise alertness, improve creativity, and prevent Parkinson's disease. However, it also raises blood pressure, aggravates stress, causes insomnia if consumed too late, and leads to addiction.[5]

▲ ENERGY BOOSTER | **Either cut out the caffeine or drink small amounts**

How much is too much coffee? A pot? A twenty-ounce venti at Starbucks? The verdict is still out, but in general, consuming more than 300 mg a day can cause jitteriness and sleeplessness. While coffee can give you a temporary get-up-and-go, drinking too much is kind of like shooting yourself in the foot: you'll give yourself a burst of energy, but eventually you'll have to pay it back. James Wyatt of Rush University Medical Center in Chicago believes our typical pattern of coffee consumption is wrong. Most people load up first thing in the morning and crash in the afternoon, when the chemical—with a half-life of up to six hours—is leaving the system. Wyatt says it's better to consume a little caffeine in the morning and continue to take it in small doses throughout the day. His subjects demonstrated no late-day crash and performed better on cognitive tests.[6] But if you need a bunch of coffee in the morning to get going, you might be addicted to caffeine, and maybe you would be better off switching to herbal tea, water, or decaffeinated drinks instead.

▲ ▲ ▲
▼ ▼ ▼

▼ ENERGY BANDIT #8 | **Insufficient intake of calcium, iron, and magnesium**

These three minerals deserve special mention because of their importance to your metabolism. They often go lacking in the adult body, particularly in older adults.

▲ ENERGY BOOSTER | **Boost your intake of these three**
important nutrients

Calcium is used to build your bones and teeth. Iron forms the basis of hemoglobin, the oxygen-transporting molecule in red blood cells. Women are especially susceptible to both calcium and iron deficiencies, due to the rigorous demands of female biology.

The mineral magnesium garners a special mention because of its importance to your energy level. Eating a balanced diet can help ensure that your vitamin and mineral needs are met. But if you still find yourself too pooped to pop, you could have a slight magnesium deficiency, says New York University nutritionist Samantha Heller, M.S., R.D. "This mineral is needed for more than 300 biochemical reactions in the body, including breaking down glucose into energy," Heller says. "So when levels are even a little low, energy can drop." In a study done at the Department of Agriculture's Human Nutrition Research Center in Grand Forks, North Dakota, women with magnesium deficiencies had higher heart rates and required more oxygen to do physical tasks than they did after their magnesium levels were restored. In essence, their bodies were working harder, which, over time, says Heller, can leave you feeling depleted. The recommended daily intake of magnesium is around 300 milligrams for women and 350 milligrams for men. Great sources of magnesium include almonds, hazelnuts, and cashews; whole grains, particularly bran cereal; and fish, especially halibut.[7]

Your body excretes excesses if it decides it doesn't need them, so there's no harm in taking iron, calcium, and magnesium supplements. Both vitamin C and copper, in moderate amounts, can aid in iron absorption; similarly, lysine and vitamin K enhance calcium absorption.

▲ ▲ ▲

Six

Pacing

Even if you do start out the day with plenty of fuel, you may eventually feel that energy slip away. You can be zipping along just fine, then—*boom!*—you hit what sports enthusiasts call "the wall." How well you handle your energy budget will determine whether you break through the wall and move on to the rest of your day—or just bounce off and slog through the mental mud.

No matter how often you might wish otherwise, you are not a robot and you can't go nonstop. That's especially true of those of you who are deskbound for most of the day. It's a simple fact that sitting at a desk for hours at a time can decrease your energy level. Occasional breaks are necessary for mental and physical health: you need to get up and stretch your legs, to get your heart pumping and your blood circulating.

However, too many rest periods can be detrimental to your productivity. If you don't have enough endurance, you'll be forced to break more frequently, and you won't get anything done. Therefore, you need to strike a balance between taking too many breaks during the day and not breaking enough, because both practices can be equally harmful. To do that, you'll need to build up your endurance and learn to pace yourself, just like a long-distance runner or mountain climber would. Think of pacing as a form of sports training for high energy.

In this chapter, you'll learn how to pace yourself appropriately. You'll discover some common causes of fatigue, and I'll suggest ways to concentrate on a task, to prevent yourself from becoming tired, and to generally improve your endurance during the day. Then you'll learn some techniques that will help bring you back to a state of alertness if your energy *does* crash. I'll show you how to physically recharge your batteries. Your mind and body will thank you for the break, and reward you with renewed energy.

▼ ▼ ▼

▼ ENERGY BANDIT #1 | Sitting down all day

When you sit all day your body can, in a sense, get bored, even if you're focused on an important task. At rest, your body needs to burn less energy to maintain itself, so there's less energy available for other things. If you don't get up occasionally, your body conserves its energy. It can be an annoying cycle: you're forced to be inactive, so you feel less and less like being active. But it's not a difficult cycle to break out of, thank goodness, as long as you're willing to change a few behaviors.

▲ ENERGY BOOSTER | Stand instead of sit

The human body is not designed to sit for hours on end. Incorporate regular physical movement into your workday, especially if most of your work is conducted at a desk:

- Stand up and take a big stretch. Clasp your hands, turn your palms toward the ceiling, and stretch upward from your tip-toes all the way through your fingertips; also stretch to the

left and right. Shrug your shoulders a few times afterward.
Then briskly scratch or massage your head.

- File a pile of papers for five minutes.
- Stand up when you take phone calls.
- Suggest stand-up meetings when you engage in short brain-storming sessions with coworkers.
- If your computer is downloading or uploading slowly, don't leave your hand by the mouse. Stand up and strike a yoga pose or stroll around the room.

▲ ▲ ▲
▼ ▼ ▼

▼ ENERGY BANDIT #2 | Working nonstop with no breaks

Failing to take breaks can affect our short-term energy and long-term health, and therefore your productivity, with everything from eye strain to carpal tunnel syndrome. Computers, like all other electronic devices, emit electromagnetic fields, as do completely natural phenomena such as the sun and lightning. Computer monitors emit an ELF, or an extremely low-frequency field; they also emit static electric fields and high-pitched sound frequencies. Extremely low frequency fields can alter neurological function, affect the pineal gland's production of melatonin, and influence dopamine. In other words, too much exposure to computers can impair your thinking ability and drain your energy level.[1]

According to Peter McLaughlin, author of *CatchFire: A 7-Step Program to Ignite Energy, Defuse Stress, and Power Boost Your Career*, 3:00 PM is "the breaking point"—the time when natural levels of energy and alertness take a nosedive.[2] While your natural rhythms are biologically based, that doesn't mean that you're a slave to your body. The body clock can be modified with the judicious application of certain behavioral tools; otherwise, certain ailments, like jet lag, would be incurable. According to McLaughlin, if you take a few minutes off from strenuous activity, your body will begin to "induce the biological changes that restore energy and strength"—even if you do absolutely nothing.[3]

▲ ENERGY BOOSTER | Give yourself a break

Otherwise intelligent people will work for hours on end without taking a break. Some people say they're so swamped, they don't have time for one. But they don't realize that taking a break would actually give them an energy boost, after which they would accomplish their tasks faster. By not taking a break, they get pulled into a black hole of energy depletion, and they end up working longer hours than if they had taken one. For some reason, we equate being unsustainably harried with being worthwhile human beings, and we feel guilty about taking breaks. We associate taking a break or relaxing with being lazy or selfish, and we equate working nonstop with having a rock-solid work ethic, being important, or maybe getting closer to that promotion. Taking a break does not make you a slacker! Rather, it makes you more productive. But not taking regular breaks will sabotage your productivity and creativity.

Don't schedule your bathroom breaks and trips to the water cooler for any specific time; go when you need to go, to help break up the monotony and to keep your body from slipping so readily into its resting metabolic rate. Then insert regular break times into your day: at mid-morning, lunchtime, mid-afternoon, and dinnertime.

▲ ▲ ▲

▼ ▼ ▼

▼ ENERGY BANDIT #3 | Not moving around enough during the day

When you're active, your muscles use the glucose fuel in your bloodstream more efficiently. Increased muscular activity means increased demand for glucose, which means that the glucose in your bloodstream won't be converted into fat. It will either be burned purely for energy, or end up incorporated into more muscle tissue, which helps you burn more energy, which makes you more energetic, which helps you build more muscle tissue . . . well, you get the picture. While it's not quite as simple as that, activity *can* trigger a nice feedback process that keeps you alert and energetic on a more continual basis.

▲ ENERGY BOOSTER | Avoid being sedentary and walk around

Don't waste your breaks by sitting down in the break room and reading the comics section of the newspaper, or by standing around the vendor area eating a doughnut. Take a brisk walk around the building. Better yet, take a brisk fifteen- to thirty-minute walk. If it's raining or severely cold, walk up and down a flight of stairs a few times instead. Your muscles will thank you for it. If you live in the city, don't make the mistake of thinking that you have to hop in the car and drive for an hour to find nature. Nature is everywhere, even in the inner city. If your company is enlightened enough to offer a walking trail down in the building's atrium, use it. If not, make do with what you've got. You can even make the fire stairs into your own StairMaster. Any of these activities can kick your body up into the physical activity energy expenditure (PAEE) phase of your metabolism.[4] At least for a while after returning from your vigorous break, you should have more energy to devote to your task.

▲ ▲ ▲
▼ ▼ ▼

▼ ENERGY BANDIT #4 | Heavy concentration

If you've been editing a book, writing code, or analyzing spreadsheets all day, the intense focus can make your energy flag. If you have low energy, these types of tasks can literally make your brain hurt.

▲ ENERGY BOOSTER | Try creative desk-energy renewal strategies

If you don't have time to take a lengthy break and have a walkabout through the office, there are still ways you can take a quick break at your desk and pump up the energy a little. If you don't have a boss (or deadline) breathing down your neck, you can close your eyes for a few minutes while remaining upright. Putting your head down on your desk is not recommended, as you're risking bad posture and the aches that go with it (or falling asleep). Other effective methods of desk-energy renewal include the following:

- Deep breathing
- Meditation
- Prayer
- Positive thinking
- Stretching
- Massaging your neck and shoulders
- A quick break to do small, routine tasks: checking your e-mail, clearing your desk, making a phone call

- Smart snacking on something that provides a nice little injection of energy: a piece of a power bar, some fruit, or a carrot stick.

All these items are minor steps to quick alertness, but they can either help you to increase your physical energy through motion or let you unwind (if only for a few minutes) from the task on which you've been concentrating. Note, however, that these are useful only when your energy is flagging and you're unable to concentrate on what you need to do. You don't want to break your focus if you're on a roll, because you'll shoot holes in your productivity.

▲ ▲ ▲
▼ ▼ ▼

▼ ENERGY BANDIT #5 | Your tasks are monotonous

We've all gotten into ruts at some point in our lives, ones that seem to take all our attention and time, all the while driving us deeper into boredom and the consequent lack of energy. Some of the things we need to do each day simply don't interest us, and it's hard to get motivated to work on them.

▲ ENERGY BOOSTER | Find an encouragement partner

If you feel stuck and unenergetic, get a friend in your office to play the "check-in game" with you. Exchange brief calls telling each other, "I'm stuck, and here's what I need to do. Can I check in with you every few hours until I start to be productive again?" Your friend may very well need something to spur him or her into activity too, so this can be a good exchange for both of you. Cleaning up your work space, working on another task, and playing music that you enjoy are also great ways to break out of a rut. Or bribe yourself with a reward when you reach that next goal—maybe a Hershey's Kiss from the candy jar, or a trip to the soda machine, or a quick leg-stretching walk around the building. The promise of a little bribe, whatever it is, helps move you along that little bit further, so you accomplish that much more before you take a break. There's no shame in that, because it helps you build your energy endurance.

Also, stave off boredom while you work. Our hobbies and interests outside of work help keep us sane. Injecting the things you're interested in into your day can help you maintain the alertness and energy levels you need to get things done. If you're a music fan, listen to some sprightly opera or interesting jazz on a Walkman or iPod as you work; think of it as a soundtrack to your life. You can also keep little reminders of the things you love (like your pets) on your desk, or take the occasional minute to chat with a fellow aficionado about a shared hobby or interest. It doesn't have to be much to keep your mind engaged and to help keep you from sliding into an energy rut. This doesn't mean you should waste inordinate amounts of time devoted to personal things; it simply means you're human and need a psychological boost occasionally by thinking about things that give you joy. I like to dash off an e-mail to a girlfriend and put some plans in place for the weekend, which gives me something to look forward to, and also gives me a refreshed burst of energy for my daily tasks.

▼ ENERGY BANDIT #6 | Slouching

The connection between your posture and your energy level might not seem immediately apparent. But if you're slumped over your desk all day, typing or reading, you're stressing your musculature and skeleton. Physical stress can have an effect on your personal energy level, and if you get a crick in your back, your productivity is certainly going to suffer. This is especially so when you sit for prolonged periods, fixated on your screen. According to scientific studies,[5] maintaining upright posture uses only a little more energy than lying down does, and much less than other forms of posture do. It's possible that this is one of the reasons why humans are bipedal.

▲ ENERGY BOOSTER | Watch your posture

In recent years we've all become a lot more aware of the value of decent ergonomic furniture. The proper desk chair and a good wrist pad, among other more esoteric items, can help you maintain the proper posture for longer periods of time, thus avoiding the everyday aches and pains that will shrink your attention span and suck away your energy. The more pain you're in, the harder you have to work to not think about it and focus on your task, drawing away more energy than would have been necessary. Right now—this very second—where do you hurt? Were you even aware of it until I mentioned it?

▼ ENERGY BANDIT #7 | Using up too much energy too soon

If you feel great every morning but you're dead by early afternoon, then you're obviously using up your energy too soon. Effective energy usage is a matter of pacing, which comes down to planning. Energy is something that should be optimized, not maximized. For example, delivering higher levels of energy to a lightbulb will not make it brighter; it will make it explode. More energy is not always better.

Think of your day's energy as a rack of wood set aside for the fireplace. It's possible to pile it all together at once and make a huge, rip-roaring bonfire that's alive with light and heat—but a few hours later, it's nothing but embers and ashes, and you'll need more wood if you want to keep it going. But if you start a small fire in the morning and carefully feed in the logs one at a time, you'll have enough wood to keep going until the late evening. So, what sounds better: a blaze of glory, or a slow, steady fire? You end up with the same amount of energy and ash, but you can do a lot more work over a longer period with the slow, steady fire.

▲ ENERGY BOOSTER | **Pace yourself**

Remember, you're not a machine. Don't squander your energy early in the day, or you'll fade by mid-afternoon. You need to take occasional breaks and work intensely for shorter periods of time; this is effective in everything from creative activity and office work to fitness training. According to executive trainers Jim Loehr and Tony Schwartz, "Managing energy, not time, is the key to high performance and personal renewal." In fact, they made that the subtitle of their book, *The Power of Full Engagement*. They emphasize that rest, not just hard work, is important to achieving anything of consequence in a decent amount of time. Basically, they preach the value of the cycle of energy management, in which you're fully engaged and focused on your work for a relatively short period of time, followed by an intense period of recovery in which you're fully disengaged and seeking renewal.[6] Many of the world's greatest leaders have been fully aware of the need for this kind of creative pacing. If Winston Churchill was able to cope during World War II by taking regular naps, then you ought to be able to do something similar.

▲ ▲ ▲

▼ ▼ ▼

Daily biological cycles

We discussed the body clock in chapter 1 as it relates to sleep. But the body clock also plays an important function during the day. It's an indisputable fact that living things undergo cyclical phenomena in most of their bodily systems, including their energy. Variously known as biological rhythms[7] and chronobiology, these phases may be long-term—as in annual migrations or menstrual cycles—or of shorter duration: for example, the ninety-minute REM cycle during sleep, or the three-hour growth-hormone cycle.

You're susceptible to circadian rhythms, which are biological patterns controlled by sunlight and temperature. This explains why newcomers to the Arctic Circle have problems adjusting to twenty-four hours of sunlight in the summer and twenty-four hours of darkness in the winter. Jet lag can similarly screw up your body clock. Why? Because humans, like flowers, insects, and bushy-tailed squirrels, are products of our environments. At the genetic level, biological rhythms are controlled by so-called "clock genes." Disruptions to the clock genes can result in out-of-whack body rhythms, such as the oddball sleep/wake cycles suffered by many victims of bipolar disorder.[8]

▲ ENERGY BOOSTER | **Respect your chronobiology**

No matter what you do, you're going to go through energy cycles during the day. Our circadian rhythms also have shorter ultradian rhythms that occur throughout the day; they are characterized by ninety-minute peaks of energy followed by ten- to twenty-minute slumps. After ninety minutes of focused activity, you're likely to suffer a loss of stamina; your energy level and alertness dip into negative territory, and suddenly you're ready for a nap. Your best bet is to understand this pattern and stop fighting it and trying to "work through it."

If you're scraping the bottom of your energy barrel, whether it's 10:00 AM or 3:00 PM, don't ignore it, because it won't get better by itself. Take a break or a nap, or do something else to bring you back to a state of alertness. Trying to concentrate on numbers, brainstorm solutions to a project, or be creative are particularly fruitless during this time. The quality of your results will be low, it will take forever, and you might have to rework mistakes later. Instead, call a friend, get a drink of water, play a quick game of solitaire on the computer, or water the plants. You may discover that a few minutes off might be just the thing you need to revamp your energy level.

▲ ▲ ▲

Seven

Health

It hurts when I do this

When you don't feel well, you have lower energy, and it's hard to be productive at home or at work. In this chapter, you will take personal responsibility for taking care of any health problems you suffer. What wellness issues are affecting your energy and causing you to feel poorly? It's important to take good care of your health, get regular checkups, and investigate seemingly chronic conditions you've resigned yourself to.

It's purely awful to feel tired all the time, but establishing the exact cause is tricky because there are so many things that could make you feel low. Don't wait for something to feel "wrong" before you get it checked out. Even if it's been years since you've investigated treatment, a lot can change and different options may now be available.

▼ ▼ ▼

▼ ENERGY BANDIT #1 | **Practicing poor self-care**

You don't go to the doctor. You haven't had your routine exams and checkups. You don't take care of your teeth. You don't spend enough time pampering yourself. If you don't take care of yourself, your ability to take care of others will decline. Have you been vigilant about getting your physical exams, dental cleanings, and vision screenings? Do you see the dermatologist right away when a mole looks even slightly suspicious, or do you put it off until you have more serious problems? Do you wonder about that mysterious pain but hope it will go away, since you don't have time to go to the doctor? You certainly don't want to expend any energy thinking about a nagging problem, let alone waste very real levels of energy if you were forced to fight a truly debilitating—and avoidable—illness.

▲ ENERGY BOOSTER | **Line up your routine checkups, screenings, and exams**

When did you last have a physical? Schedule future reminders on your calendar for the following:

- Physical screenings and blood work, which vary by gender and age. Men need an annual prostate exam and a colonoscopy over age fifty. Women need an annual gynecological exam and a mammogram over age forty (consider the new digital mammogram, which exposes you to less radiation than film X-rays).
- Screenings for specific illnesses and diseases where there's a family history
- Complete blood workup (hormone levels, cholesterol, blood glucose, thyroid, vitamins). If you feel sluggish even after a good night's rest, get a blood test for thyroid function and anemia. It won't give you an instant boost, but if this proves to be your problem, getting medication will soon have you back up to speed. If indeed you have anemia, your body isn't getting the amount of oxygen you need to sustain energy, due to a reduction of red blood cells.
- Dermatological exam for any suspicious moles (annually)

- Dental exam (be sure to point out any red, black, or white spots on the gums, which could be potentially cancerous)
- Vision screening

Don't forget to keep good records. What was the exact name of that antibiotic that caused an allergic reaction two years ago? Do you know your eyeglass prescription? If you're counting on your doctor to have the facts, you may be out of luck if you change doctors or haven't seen that physician in a few years. Whenever a specialist writes to your primary-care physician, ask to be copied. While you're at it, gather your family's medical history so you can help your physician reduce your risk of problems and pinpoint your symptoms. You may want to buy computer software that tracks this information electronically, such as HealthFile Lite or HealthFile Plus (twenty dollars and thirty dollars, www.wakefieldsoft.com/healthfile). Contact your doctors, past and present, and ask for copies of your files, including the following:

- Lab results
- Imaging studies
- Immunization records
- Prescriptions and doses

▲ ▲ ▲
▼ ▼ ▼

▼ ENERGY BANDIT #2 | **Poor dental hygiene**

Every year more than 3 million miles of dental floss are sold in the United States. That's a lot, but the total should be much higher, since that amount works out to only about one flossing per week for the average American.

▲ ENERGY BOOSTER | Take good care of your teeth

Flossing your choppers once a day can potentially add years to your life. If you don't floss, you could develop gum disease. Studies from the American Academy of Periodontology suggest that when the gums are infected, periodontal bacteria by-products can enter the bloodstream and travel to major organs, setting off other problems. Research suggests this may contribute to the development of heart disease, the nation's leading cause of death (people with periodontal disease are almost twice as likely to suffer from coronary artery disease as those with healthy teeth and gums); increase the risk of stroke; increase a woman's risk of having a preterm low-birth-weight baby; and pose a serious threat to people whose health is compromised by diabetes, respiratory disease, or osteoporosis.[1] Not taking proper care of your teeth can literally make you sick. With illness comes low energy. You must learn to love your teeth. You could decide you're going to floss every day this month. If you hate using dental floss, try my favorite flosser, the Reach Access Flosser, www.reachaccess.com. Keep it in your toothbrush holder as a daily reminder to floss.

How about your toothbrush? How long has it been since you've purchased a new one? If you use a manual toothbrush, replace it every three months. When you open a new one, use a permanent marker to label the handle with the brush's expiration date. Or perhaps your action today will be to purchase an electric toothbrush, which is worth the investment. The last time I went for a checkup and cleaning, the hygienist commented, "You must use an electric toothbrush." "How can you tell?" I asked. "Because your gums are very healthy, and you don't have any tarter or plaque buildup," she replied. I like the Sonicare Elite e9000 series, www.sonicare.com. Don't forget to replace the heads frequently.

▲ ▲ ▲

▼ ▼ ▼

The common cold

Having a cold makes you miserable and saps your energy. Many times sick coworkers show up for work anyway—a phenomenon commonly called presenteeism. AdvancePCS, a health-services company based in Irving, Texas, estimates that presenteeism is responsible for two-thirds of the $250 billion lost in health-related costs in the United States every year.[2] If you notice that someone at work is coughing, sneezing, or sniffling, avoid touching things after that person does and keep your distance. If you're sick, stay at home so that you don't transmit your illness to others.

▲ ENERGY BOOSTER | **Treat your cold symptoms**

- If you do catch a cold, do not beg your doctor for antibiotics, which are not effective against viral infections. There is something you can do, however. Research conducted by the Cleveland Clinic Foundation, one of the world's largest and most prestigious health centers, confirms the efficacy of Zicam (www.zicam.com). This clinical study demonstrated that Zicam reduced the severity and duration of common-cold symptoms even when treatment was started as late as the second day after the onset of illness. The study appeared in the January 2003 issue of *QJM: An International Journal of Medicine.*[3]
- If your congestion, headache, and fever continue for two weeks or longer, you may have developed a sinus or ear infection, in which case you would need to see your doctor for an antibiotic.
- A study published in the November 21, 2002, issue of the *American Journal of Therapeutics* shows that taking zinc

lozenges on a daily basis can significantly reduce the possibility of getting a cold. The study, involving 378 subjects at a high school for over a total of 170,000 patient days, showed that the incidence of colds was reduced by as much as 62 percent.[4]

▲ ▲ ▲
▼ ▼ ▼

▼ ENERGY BANDIT #4 | A weak immune system from an infection

Certain viruses, like mononucleosis (also called glandular fever) and the flu virus, are often accompanied by exhaustion, sore throat, headaches, and swollen tonsils and/or lymph nodes. Even when the virus has run its course after a couple of weeks, your body is left in a very vulnerable state. It's almost as if your body becomes programmed to have an intense response to every little virus in the future, knocking you back to feeling exhausted and vulnerable again and again. If you've had a serious virus recently, you'll have to take additional steps to stay healthy.

▲ ENERGY BOOSTER | Disinfect your environment

In addition to getting a flu shot, avoid getting sick by keeping your environment germ-free. Wipe your desk surfaces on a regular basis: touching your desk and eating at your desk cause a buildup of bacteria. According to research from the University of Arizona in Tucson, the average desk has one hundred times more bacteria than your kitchen table and four hundred times more than the average toilet. The top five most germ-contaminated spots were (in order): phone, desktop, water-fountain handle, microwave-door handle, and keyboard.[5] Use Lysol spray on phone receivers and keyboards.

Many people (disgustingly) do not wash their hands after using the restroom, so door handles can transmit viruses and bacteria. In a restroom, dry your hands off with a paper towel, and then open the door with it before tossing. If you sign into a register at the front desk, use your own pen. Someone may have coughed into his/her hand and then used that pen right before you. When you think of all the common things that people touch in your workplace—the coffee pot, the fax machine, the copy machine—it becomes one big petri dish. I'm not suggesting you be paranoid, but be aware and careful. Wash your hands frequently with warm water and soap, and don't put your hands to your face.

▲ ▲ ▲
▼ ▼ ▼

▼ ENERGY BANDIT #5 | High cortisol levels and hormonal imbalance

Symptoms such as fatigue, irritability, hot flashes, and night sweats can point to a hormone imbalance. In menopausal women, the hormones progesterone and estrogen can be out of whack, which can cause low energy and general misery. In men, hormone imbalances include androgen excess and testosterone deficiencies. But a lesser-known hormonal problem is cortisol imbalance. When you're stressed, worried, or tense, your adrenal glands produce four neuro-transmitters (or stress-managing chemicals): epinephrine, norepi-nephrine, cortisol, and DHEA. In the right amounts, these chemicals will help you stay healthy. But when you're under stress on a regular basis, your adrenal glands become overtaxed. Then, instead of pro-tecting you from stress, they produce too much of these chemicals, leaving you exhausted, mentally drained, and irritable.

▲ ENERGY BOOSTER | **Have more sex**

Spending quality time between the sheets once or twice a week can lower your stress and improve your immune system; orgasms may relieve headaches and menstrual symptoms. People with a good sex life also seem better able to ward off colds and depression and might even gain protection from heart disease, says Barbara Bartlik, a psychiatrist and sex therapist at the New York Weill Cornell Medical Center.[6] Sex also has many of the same cardiovascular benefits as aerobics. Having intimate relations boosts the production of life-lengthening hormones; people with healthy sexual relationships, in fact, live longer. Even cuddling is beneficial: touching releases oxytocin, the hormone associated with emotional closeness.

▼ ENERGY BANDIT #6 | **Forgetting that laughter is the best medicine**

If you get sick a lot, perhaps you're just not laughing enough. Laughing can build levels of the antibody IgA, the body's first line of defense against germs, says Carl Charnetski, Ph.D., a psychology professor at Wilkes University, in Wilkes-Barre, Pennsylvania, as quoted in *Shape* magazine in December 2006.

▲ ENERGY BOOSTER | **Laugh!**

Numerous studies have been conducted on the health benefits of laughter. Drs. Lee Berk and Stanley Tan of the Loma Linda University Medical Centre in California studied volunteers watching funny videos. They analyzed blood samples and found that laughter lowers cortisol and increases endorphins—the opposite of the effects of stress. While stress creates high levels of cortisol that suppress the immune system, laughter increases your T cells, which attack viruses, and natural killer cells, which attack cancer cells. In another study, researchers at Indiana State University compared women who laughed out loud at funny films to women watching a boring tourism video. Bottom line: The immune systems of the people who laughed out loud were increased by up to 40 percent compared to those who were watching the tourism film. Generally speaking, laughing counters the negative effects of stress, which can include anxiety, depression, high blood pressure, heart disease, and insomnia, just to name a few. Laughter controls high blood pressure and heart disease by reducing the release of stress-inducing hormones. It releases endorphins, the body's feel-good painkillers; it also boosts production of serotonin, the body's natural antidepressant. Laughter also provides an internal massage for the intestines, liver, spleen, kidneys, and adrenal glands; the adrenal glands are a key organ regulating energy levels. Laughter even reduces snoring by exercising the soft palate and throat.[7]

▼ ENERGY BANDIT #7 | Consistent physical pain

It's hard to do much of anything when you're in pain. Chronic pain can really sap your energy. Like many people, I'm guilty of putting up with too much pain, deciding "that's just the way it is; nothing I can do about it." Don't suffer silently with symptoms. Brainstorm your top five most significant health problems (headache, high blood pressure, toothache, insomnia, allergies, pain, asthma, hoarseness, acne, foot pain, constipation, joint problems, sinus problems, hair loss, heartburn, and so forth). How would you like to feel instead?

▲ ENERGY BOOSTER | Don't give up on fighting chronic pain

About a year ago, my lower back started hurting. I ignored it, assuming it had to do with some old car accidents. Then, several months ago, I bent over to blow-dry my hair and—*bam*—my lower back went out. I went to my knees with the most excruciating pain I've ever felt (except perhaps childbirth). I hobbled to the doctor like a very old woman, all bent over, and he injected my back with an anti-inflammatory, gave me pain medication, and told me to come back for an X-ray when I recovered. Obediently, I returned a week later for the X-ray. Diagnosis: degenerative arthritis, a completely different problem from the issues with the rest of my back. He gave me some medication, exercises, and herbal remedies that have made a huge difference in the pain I feel while sitting for extended periods of time at my desk.

Take a moment to visualize what you wish to happen in the future regarding seemingly chronic health issues. Call a new doctor in a different field and get an appointment. Ask your primary-care physician for a referral. Spend some time researching on the Internet. Don't take "You'll have to live with it" as an answer. Don't make the same mistake I did and assume your pain is inevitable. Get it checked out.

▲ ▲ ▲
▼ ▼ ▼

▼ ENERGY BANDIT #8 | Allergies

When I was in my twenties, I developed an extreme allergic reaction to my cats and was saddened to have to give them away. Although I'd never had allergies as a child, I suddenly couldn't tolerate most animals with fur, along with myriad trees, grass, dust, and weeds. The next ten years were filled with nasal sprays, antihistamines, eye drops, and inhalers. Just feeling normal was difficult, and

I resigned myself to taking these medications for the rest of my life. Years later, a friend told me her child was getting allergy shots. I'd never heard of that. I investigated the shots with a new allergist and started receiving injections. To my delight, two years later, I was symptom-free and drug-free. I became immune to the point that I once again have a pet—a bichon frisé, a low-allergen breed of dog—with no adverse reactions.

Even if you didn't have allergies as a child, everyday irritants such as exercise, cold air, and car exhaust can cause problems at any age. You can develop asthma even as an adult, so if you have a cough that lasts longer than a few weeks, you may need to visit an allergist to get a lung-function test (find one in your area at www.AAAAI .org).

▲ ENERGY BOOSTER | **Clean your air**

If you don't have seasonal allergies or pets, but you're sneezing a lot, your nose is running, and your eyes are watering, call an air-duct and furnace cleaning company. They will inspect, clean, vacuum, and service your air ducts and cooling and heating systems. A buildup of mold can aggravate allergies and asthma. A buildup of debris and/or soot in your chimney not only can cause fires but also can raise your odds of carbon monoxide poisoning. Change the batteries in your smoke and carbon monoxide detectors. The Environmental Protection Agency says the air you breathe inside your home can be ten times as polluted as the air outside! Concentrations of volatile organic compounds (VOCs), such as paints and lacquers; paint strippers; cleaning supplies; pesticides; building materials and furnishings; office equipment such as copiers and printers, correction fluids, and carbonless copy paper; and graphics and craft materials, including glues and adhesives, permanent markers, and photographic solutions, can be two to five times higher inside homes than outside.[8]

When my son James developed chronic ear infections as a baby and had to have surgery to remove his adenoids, we purchased a HEPA (High Efficiency Particle Arrestor) air cleaner for his bedroom, which captures most common household allergens such as dust, mold spores, and pet dander. We saw a marked improvement in his allergy symptoms after a few weeks.

▲ ▲ ▲

Part Two
PRACTICES

Eight

Quick Fixes

You eat well, you get enough sleep, you exercise every day, but your energy is at rock-bottom. Maybe it's toward the end of the workday. Maybe it's the end of the week. Maybe it's a new moon. Maybe it's the first day of your menstrual cycle. Maybe your biorhythm cycle is at its natural ebb. Maybe it's the dead of winter and any sane mammal would be hibernating instead of driving to work at 7:00 AM while it's still dark outside. These quick little fixes come in very handy in such situations. I'll show you how to open your mind and get out the door, how to take a deep breath and strike a pose, and how to act like a kid and laugh till it hurts. These tricks also come in handy for an energy boost during your mid-afternoon break or when you're trying to get off the caffeine roller coaster.

▼ ▼ ▼

▼ ENERGY BANDIT #1 | **Staring at a computer all day**

You've probably seen cartoons that show a stooped-over ape evolving into an upright human, which devolves into a human form stooped over a computer at a desk! With all the televisions, remote controls, computers, and video games in today's world, we have become incredibly sedentary. And lack of movement translates to lack of energy. A 1997 National Health Interview Survey found that a whopping 40 percent of U.S. adults *never* engage in any physically active activities whatsoever during leisure time, such as exercise or sports. A sedentary lifestyle is a risk factor for coronary heart disease, hypertension, colon cancer, and diabetes.[1] When you take breaks throughout the day, get away from the computer. And even when you're at the office, you can interject physical movement into desk work.

▲ ENERGY BOOSTER | **Recharge regularly**

Get the most mileage from your mid-morning, lunchtime, mid-afternoon, and dinnertime breaks with little tricks:

- Brush, floss, and/or use a mouthwash rinse on your teeth.
- Pat a cool, dampened paper towel or washcloth all over your face and neck, especially around your eyes. You can also use a moistened cotton swab around your eyes. If you work at home, take a shower. Sprinkle eucalyptus on the shower floor, stand under steaming hot water, rub your body all over with a loofah, and then blast yourself with a shot of cold water.
- Jump-start your brain and body back into maximum efficiency by doing something that gives you a jolt: eating an Atomic Fireball, drinking a glass of tart lemonade, standing in front of the air conditioner, or giving your scalp a brisk rub.
- Stave off dehydration. Stand up and chug as much water as your stomach can hold. You'll soon have to go to the restroom, which will force you to take another break.
- Feed the fish. Watch them swim for a few minutes; the sound and motion of water are naturally relaxing for human beings, whose bodies are 70 percent water.

- Water the plants. You don't have a plant in your office? Get one! A study conducted by the Washington State University College of Agriculture found that indoor plants reduce stress and increase productivity. Researchers found that productivity and reaction time increased by 12 percent when workers performed computer tasks in offices with indoor plants as compared to those without plants.[2]

▲ ▲ ▲
▼ ▼ ▼

▼ ENERGY BANDIT #2 | A lack of fresh air and sunshine

The human body's 100 trillion cells require a constant supply of oxygen. Sure, there's plenty of oxygen in your office—but it can get stale, especially in winter. Getting outside is literally a "breath of fresh air." The heart circulates blood to the lungs, exchanging carbon dioxide for fresh oxygen. Fresh oxygen improves the brain's function, boosting your energy level.

▲ ENERGY BOOSTER | Get outside and get some sunshine

All too often we overlook the profound power of a little outdoor time to boost our energy levels—not to mention our spirits. Fresh air infuses you with a sense of well-being and happiness by increasing the brain's production of serotonin. And serotonin production promotes sound sleep, an added bonus of outdoor time.[3] Human beings have a natural love of the outdoors. Environmental psychologists from the University of Michigan found in a 2004 survey that regular walkers are more likely to walk for a longer period of time if their route involves natural settings of woods, water, or plants. The researchers concluded that people who enjoy exercising outdoors also benefit from mental revitalization.[4] Likewise, a study in Copenhagen found that easily accessible green spaces such as gardens and parks decrease mental stress.[5]

For health reasons, you need about ten minutes of daily sunlight, even if it's overcast. (But don't forget the sunscreen!) Sunlight increases the brain's production of endorphins, which instills a sense of well-being and prevents depression. Sunshine also improves circulation, lowers the heart rate, and regulates blood pressure and blood sugar. It also increases metabolism and melatonin production at night, making for more sound sleep. As if that isn't enough, sunshine even converts cholesterol into vitamin D and boosts the immune system by increasing the number of white blood cells. Getting outside is important even if you keep your blinds open, because windows filter out 95 percent of beneficial light.[6]

Go for a quick walk or work in the yard for just a few minutes—sweep the deck, shovel the snow, or water some flowers. Never underestimate the power of fresh air to boost your mood, energy, and overall health. There's a reason it's called "the great outdoors." Meander through a flower garden or a park, or walk for a few blocks. Sit next to a fountain. Listen to the birds chirp. Look up to see what the clouds are doing. If you pay close enough attention, you may even spy genuine wildlife such as hawks or peregrine falcons.

▲ ▲ ▲
▼ ▼ ▼

▼ ENERGY BANDIT #3 | **Stiff, tight, sore muscles**

The more tension you have in your muscles, the less power you have. Tight muscles reduce oxygen flow, blood flow, and energy flow. Golfers will tell you that when they hit the ball with power, they are feeling relaxed. They can choke up if feeling tight and tense over the ball. Power occurs when our bodies are relaxed, not when they are stiff, tight, and rigid. Reducing tension in your muscles can help you restore energy flow.

| **Stretch at your desk**

A few simple, quick stretches at your desk will alleviate any stiffness and posture problems and put you back on a more energetic keel:

- *Fingers.* Separate and straighten your fingers until tension is felt. Hold for ten seconds.
- *Hands.* Relax your fingers, and then bend them at the knuckles into a tight fist. Hold for ten seconds, then repeat.
- *Shoulders.* Shrug your shoulders toward your ears until you feel a slight tension in your neck. Hold for five seconds, and then relax your shoulders into the normal position. Repeat two more times. This is good to use at the first sign of tightness in the shoulder and neck area.
- *Upper back.* Interlace your fingers and place them behind your head. Keep your elbows straight out to the sides while maintaining a straight upper body. Pull your shoulder blades together, as if you're trying to hold a ball between them. Hold the tension for ten seconds, and then relax. Repeat two more times. Do this when your upper back is tight.
- *Neck.* Start with your head upright and balanced. Slowly tilt your head to one side, until you feel an easy stretch. Hold this stretch without bouncing until the tension eases, about twenty seconds, being careful not to overstretch. Repeat on the other side. Do two more times on each side.
- *Neck.* Now slowly turn your head toward one shoulder, until you feel an easy stretch. Hold this stretch without bouncing until the tension eases, about twenty seconds. Do not overstretch. Repeat on the other side. Do two more times on each side.

- **Neck.** Gently tilt your head forward (never tilt your head **back)** to stretch the back of the neck. Do not stretch to the point of pain. Hold for ten seconds, and then return to normal. Repeat three to five times, until your neck feels looser.
- **Arms/upper back.** Hold your left arm just above the elbow with your right hand. Gently pull your elbow toward the opposite (right) shoulder. Look over your left shoulder. Hold the stretch for twenty seconds, and then repeat on the other side. Do two more times.
- **Arms/shoulder blades.** Interlace your fingers. With your palms facing out, straighten your elbows as you stretch your arms out in front of you. Stretch until you feel tension through the upper part of your back and shoulder blades. Hold for twenty seconds, then repeat two times.
- **Arms/upper rib cage.** Interlace your fingers. With your palms facing out, straighten your elbows as you stretch your arms above your head. Stretch until you feel tension through the upper sides of your rib cage. Hold for twenty seconds, then repeat.
- **Shoulders/triceps.** Bend your left elbow. With your right hand, gently push your upper arm up behind your head until an easy tension is felt in your triceps (upper arm). Hold for twenty seconds before switching sides. Repeat.
- **Lower back/hips.** While sitting in a chair, cross your left leg over your right leg. Rest your right elbow (or forearm) on the outside of the upper thigh of the left leg. Now apply some steady, controlled pressure against your leg as you turn to look over your left shoulder. Hold for twenty seconds, then repeat on the other side.

(*Bonus:* Send an e-mail to Stretches@TheProductivityPro.com and receive an article with photos of each stretch.)

▲ ▲ ▲

▼ ▼ ▼

▼ ENERGY BANDIT #4 | **Lack of flexibility**

Studies show that people who practice yoga exhibit lower anxiety, more efficient heart and respiratory function, better physical fitness, and are more resistant to stress. Yoga increases mental focus and alertness, stills the mind, and provides physical and emotional relaxation. It even reduces blood pressure, depression, cholesterol levels, insomnia, obesity, stress, and PMS. Yoga's focused movements coupled with steady breathing elicit the relaxation response, dissolving anxiety and promoting peace of mind.[7]

▲ ENERGY BOOSTER | **Strike a pose**

Yoga, which originated in India, has been around for thousands of years. Take off your shoes and strike an easy yet energizing yoga pose. Also take off your socks if they render the floor surface too slippery:

- **Warrior I:** Stand with your feet together. Step your left leg backward far enough that your right leg is in a lunge. Don't let your right knee extend farther forward than your right ankle. Now raise both arms overhead, palms touching. Look up at your thumbs. Stretch fully up through your fingertips. Hold for ten breaths. To release, bring your hands to your hips and step your left leg forward. Repeat with the other leg.
- **Warrior II:** Stand with your feet wide apart. Turn your right foot outward 90 degrees, and turn your left foot inward 45 degrees. Extend your arms outward from your shoulders to form a T. Bend your right knee at a 90-degree angle, but don't let it extend out over your toes. Now turn your head to look over your right arm. Stretch both arms strongly through

your fingertips. Hold for ten breaths. To release, bring your hands to your hips and step your legs back together. Repeat with the other leg. This pose will also boost confidence.

- **Standing forward bend:** Stand with your feet together. Slowly bend forward from the waist; grasp your ankles or place your palms or fingertips on the floor, whichever is most comfortable. It's fine to bend your knees slightly if necessary. Hold for ten breaths. This pose will also soothe stress.

▲ ▲ ▲
▼ ▼ ▼

▼ ENERGY BANDIT #5 | Taking life too seriously

Don't fall into the trap of taking yourself, your job, and your life too seriously. Don't let your problems seem bigger than they really are. Take time to laugh, be silly, and act like a kid. Silliness is an art form, a stress buster, and an energy-boosting shot in the arm. Laughter enriches the blood with oxygen and increases stamina through a higher oxygen supply. So get in touch with your inner child. You're never too old to have a happy childhood—or to boost your energy in fun and unusual ways! Just five minutes of acting like a kid will absolutely skyrocket your energy level.

▲ ENERGY BOOSTER | Engage in some silliness

- Play a nose flute. You can order them in bright, fun colors from the Nash Company at http://www.nashco.com/noseflutes.html. Hold it up to your mouth and nose. Open your mouth, but close your glottis by inhaling and exhaling only through your nose while keeping your mouth open. Play a silly tune, such as the *Wallace and Gromit* theme song, the Warner Brothers Looney Tunes theme song, or "The Purple

People Eater." Pass some out to your coworkers and encourage them to take a silliness break with you. I first learned of these from my buddy Tim Gard (www.timgard.com), and they are a hit with his audiences and my own kids.

- Tell a coworker a clean joke.
- Subscribe to *Funny Times*: 888-386-6984, www.funny times.com.
- Read a *Calvin and Hobbes* comic book during your morning "reading" time.
- Play limericks with five people around a table. Each person has a small piece of paper and a pen, and writes one line of a limerick. After writing one line, you pass it to the person on your left. You continue thus writing a line and passing it to the left until you have five five-line limericks. After the last line is completed, you pass it to the left once again, and then everyone takes turns reading the limerick they're holding.
- Color! Who says coloring with crayons or markers is just for kids? Tap your inherent creativity and fun. While you're at it, get out the glitter, scissors, and construction paper.
- Infuse a little fun and silliness into your walk in the park! Skip. Swing. Few simple activities are more exhilarating than swinging. Feel that silly giddiness in your belly when you're at the peak of your forward movement. Tilt your head backward to watch the world from a new perspective.
- Jump on the merry-go-round. You will giggle helplessly as centrifugal force makes your all-too-serious world spin out of control.
- Catch snowflakes on your tongue.
- Plop backward into the snow and make a snow angel.

▲ ▲ ▲

▼ ▼ ▼

| Sluggish senses

Just as an alarm clock and bright light stimulate your senses and wake you up in the morning, sometimes your senses need to be awakened during the day. Maybe you're experiencing that postlunch coma and need to give your senses a blast of bracing energy.

▲ ENERGY BOOSTER | Follow your nose with some aromatherapy

Keep bottles of scented oils by your desk; uncap and sniff as needed. Be wary of synthetically scented candles and incense. Instead, use all-natural essential oils to avoid sneezing; besides, coworkers may be sensitive to perfumes and scents.

- If you're irritable or fatigued, dab some lavender oil behind your ears and on the insides of your wrists, and then run your fingers through your hair. Lavender is calming and soothing.
- Other invigorating essential oils include lemon, lemon balm, juniper, orange, and spearmint.
- Likewise, invigorate yourself with peppermint oil if your energy level is at rock-bottom—but don't use different types of essential oils simultaneously. Be sure to wash your hands after applying peppermint oil, as it's not fun if you get it in your eyes.
- To sustain energy after work, plug a car diffuser sprinkled with oil into the cigarette lighter, or put a few drops on the air-conditioning or defrost vents and turn on the fan.

▲ ▲ ▲

▾ ▾ ▾

▾ ENERGY BANDIT #7 | **Modern-world burnout**

Many people think that alternative healing therapies are corny, though they've withstood the test of time for thousands of years and are now being confirmed by Western medicine.

▲ ENERGY BOOSTER | **Try some ancient exercises**

Be willing to try something new:

- Give yourself an ear rub. Traditional Chinese medicine considers the ear to be a microcosm of the entire body; so when you stimulate your ears, you are invigorating all internal organs and systems. Cup your hands over your ears and rub them vigorously until they are red and warm.[8] The ears are also directly related to the kidney meridian, which is directly related to energy levels.
- Relieve the pressure with some acupressure. Acupressure was developed in China five thousand years ago; it is the simplest and oldest form of human medicine. There are more than six hundred acupressure points in the human body, and they lie along the body's fourteen primary meridians, or energy channels. Western science has confirmed the existence of meridians with sensitive electrical devices. Acupressure releases endorphins, the body's natural painkillers, which are one thousand times more powerful than morphine! Press the acupressure point called ST36, which is also referred to as Three Mile Point because it gives marathon runners such an incredible energy boost, they can run for another three miles! This acupressure point is four finger widths below your kneecap, and one fin-

ger width outside the shinbone; it lies on the muscle that flexes when you move your foot upward and downward.[9] Another good one is on your hand, between the thumb and forefinger (the web). Or on the bottom of your feet, moving up and down the soles.

- Breathe—just breathe. Sit in a comfortable position and close your eyes. Inhale and exhale deeply through your nose like you are smelling a rose. Part your teeth slightly and place the tip of your tongue at the top rear of your upper teeth, where the roof of your mouth meets your teeth. When thoughts arise, let them gently float past without getting caught up in them. This is harder than it sounds. But don't chastise yourself for thoughts popping up; if you're alive, it's going to happen. Stare at the designs on the insides of your eyelids. Or focus your mind on your breath. Or count in your mind; whenever a thought pops into your head, start all over again with the number 1. You can also repeat a meaningful word or phrase over and over in your mind, such as "calm-ness within" or "I am energized." This chanting is called tran-scendental meditation, or TM for short. Studies show that the body achieves a deeper state of relaxation during TM than during ordinary rest. TM increases intelligence, perception, and creativity; electroencephalograms chart a heightened state of mental coherence and alertness. TM has even been shown to decrease high blood pressure and illness rates by more than 50 percent![10] Blow out through your mouth as if you're blowing out birthday candles.

▲ ▲ ▲

▼ ▼ ▼

▼ ENERGY BANDIT #8 | Being uncomfortable in your clothes

There's a reason casual Friday was invented—it's because we finally followed our intuition that uncomfortable clothing restricts our energy flow! In the eighties movie *Tootsie*, Dustin Hoffman dresses up as a woman to get a job. While he's donning women's apparel he says something akin to "Who's the @#!! who invented high heels?!" Wearing high heels on a regular basis can cause serious foot problems, such as hammertoes, bunions, corns, calluses, Achilles problems, and even stress fractures.[11] And that's just your feet! High heels also cause lower-back problems, poor posture, spinal misalignment, and knee osteoarthritis; they place abnormal stress on the front and back of the knee, increasing pressure by 22 to 26 percent. Although wide heels are slightly better for your feet, they're just as bad for your knees.[12]

▲ ENERGY BOOSTER | Feel good in your skin

- Some people believe that the more hours a woman wears a bra, the higher her chances are of developing breast cancer because bras restrict circulation throughout the lymph system.[13] If you work in a home office, go braless occasionally.
- Wear comfortable dress shoes. Save high heels for special occasions—such as attending an evening function.
- Don't wear a tie. My husband will attest that wearing a suit jacket when it is 90 degrees outside is nothing short of torture. Try going without a tie; just wear an oxford shirt with a suit jacket if you need to be more presentable for a meeting.
- Dress for success. This doesn't necessarily mean wearing constrictive clothing such as high heels that will zap your energy in ten minutes flat. Dress comfortably, but dress to impress.

Your body's energy needs to be able to flow. When you look good, others respect and admire you, and it boosts your confidence and energy.

- Wear your favorite "power suit." We all have an outfit that makes us look like a million bucks and boosts our confidence. Wear it on days when you need to be especially energetic.
- Color your clothing. Instead of boring gray or black, wear bold colors such as red or orange. Just looking at yourself in a mirror can give you a lift when you feel lethargic.

▲ ▲ ▲

Nine

Relaxation

Practices quiz item #9:
I am the master of the universe!

While chapter 6, on Pacing, deals primarily with the time you spend at work, this chapter deals with your free time. We'll discuss how leisure activities and relaxation can reduce your stress levels and increase your energy. We'll chat about the benefits of reading, talking, playing games, and other nongadget pastimes. Even these seemingly quiet, relaxing uses of free time are energy builders—not energy drains.

▼ ▼ ▼

▼ ENERGY BANDIT #1 | **Getting caught up in a major production**

If you have recently undergone a particularly busy spell, you may get addicted to going full-throttle 24-7. If you've ever planned a major special event, wedding, or conference, you know exactly what I'm talking about. You eat, sleep, and breathe the event planning for a very long time—handling everything from the keynote speaker's travel arrangements to a seating chart for four hundred people to centerpieces. Once the event is over, you're ready to get off the treadmill, but you just keep going round and round. It's as if you don't know what to do with yourself; you can't "come down" off your high. The very same thing can happen in shorter time periods too, whether it's one day, one week, or one month. You have to recognize when you're stuck in "on" mode and gently switch yourself to "off."

▲ ENERGY BOOSTER | **Step off the merry-go-round**

When your mind is sick and tired of working, but your body can't stop, the first step—and it's a tricky one—is to realize the disconnection between those two situations. If you're going 90 mph all day every day, but all you can think about is relaxing or "making it all stop," that's your signal. Other signals include tightness in your chest, lashing out at everyone within a five-mile radius for having the audacity even to look at you, crying at the drop of a hat, or thinking that you'll actually get to the end of your to-do list if you do just this "one more thing." Act on it. Slam on the brakes.

Perhaps you're so used to spending most of your time doing something that you don't know how to relax. Here are some suggestions:

- Stop spending every waking moment of your life doing something related to work, the kids, or running the household. Let the housework go for a few days. Don't waste any free time that comes your way "catching up" on domestic duties. Don't even *think* about using your free time to run the vacuum cleaner.
- Notice the world around you. Go watch the sun set from your porch swing. If you're pumping gas, decide not to haul out your cell phone and instead just notice every detail around you for two minutes. What kind of flowers are growing on the median? How does the breeze feel? Stop the daily blur that is your life.
- Accept the help and caregiving of others. Get over yourself.

You're not a superhero. Cash in that rain check for a back rub from your spouse. When the clouds open, the sun gleams, and your teenager says the most amazing thing—"Do you need me to do anything?"—by all means, take him up on it.

- Go out to eat. Just getting out of the rut of cooking, eating, and cleaning up the same old stuff at home can make you feel rejuvenated in no time. It's so nice to be waited on for a change.

- Engage in a little recreational time, especially of the entertainment sort. Go see a movie (a really funny one). Go to a comedy club. Go see a funny play. Go dancing.

▲ ▲ ▲
▼ ▼ ▼

▼ ENERGY BANDIT #2 | Feeling guilty about relaxing

We all need to stop and smell the roses on a regular basis, but for some odd reason, we feel guilty about a little R&R. This can be particularly true of women, especially mothers, including those who work outside the home. Women often feel obligated to take care of everyone else. They bring home the bacon, fry it up in a pan, help Johnny with homework, wash a load of dirty soccer uniforms, bake cookies for tomorrow's class party, and finally collapse into bed at 11:30 PM. But guess what? No one's head is going to burst into flames if you take a hot bath. Your household and your life are not going to fall apart if you take a few minutes to take care of yourself. Having a strong work ethic can also make us feel guilty about relaxing. Here in the West, we're firmly entrenched in the forty-hour-plus workweek. And within our society, certain geographic locations embrace a strong work ethic quite emphatically, such as in the Midwest. But did you know that working fewer than forty hours a week does not make you a less important or less impressive human being? Really. It does not render you a slacker.

▲ ENERGY BOOSTER | Understand that rest is not a bad thing

Do you feel guilty about going to the bathroom? Do you feel guilty about eating? Sleeping? Having a roof over your head? Of course not! That's because these things are basic necessities. And just like all these, relaxation is a *basic necessity*! Do you plug in your rechargeable batteries? Your laptop? Your digital camera? You are a giant, walking rechargeable battery. You have to regularly stop to recharge yourself, or you'll slowly wilt into the lifeless zone. Even God kicked back on the seventh day! Rest is a natural and necessary phenomenon. Day turns to night. Fall turns to winter. The moon wanes. Animals hibernate in winter. Have you ever noticed squirrels taking breaks from gathering nuts and lounging on tree branches on hot summer days? Trees and perennial plants sleep in the winter. Even the sun takes regular breaks to let a little darkness fall. You exist in harmony with nature and need leisure too. Finding time to rest, without guilt, will recharge your batteries and ensure higher results than if you worked nonstop. If your spouse takes your child to a birthday party, and you find yourself with two hours of alone time, don't succumb to chores and laundry. You aren't "wasting" the time if you do something for yourself. You do not have to be productive every minute of your life.

▲ ▲ ▲
▼ ▼ ▼

▼ ENERGY BANDIT #3 | Never taking time for yourself

It is okay to think about yourself and do something simply for the pleasure of it. I put a "Laura play day" on my calendar every month. I spend the day doing things I love, just for me: massage, manicure, pedicure, lunch with a girlfriend. It's not about being selfish; it's about self-care and energy replenishment.

▲ ENERGY BOOSTER | **Set aside "me" time regularly**

Remember the Calgon bath crystals commercial from the seventies? "Calgon, take me away!" Pamper yourself. It never hurts to indulge yourself on occasion. Everyone needs a little "me" time, so set some aside every day. This should be time *outside* of playing with the kids; luxuriate in this time after the kids are in bed. If you have no choice but to enjoy "me" time when the kids are awake, draw firm, healthy boundaries with family members about not disturbing you. Here are some things you could do during "me" time:

- Enjoy your favorite creative hobby, whatever that may be: Do woodworking. Draw. Paint. Play guitar. Sing. Knit. Make crafts. Paint ceramics. Write in your journal. Take photos. Work on your scrapbook.
- Indulge in some fun: Go fishing. Go golfing. Dance to upbeat music. Garden. Play tennis. Play volleyball. Shoot some hoops.
- Luxuriate in relaxation: Read. Take a long, hot bath. Meditate. Do yoga. Stretch.
- Stop planning. The next time you have a Saturday morning with nothing on the calendar, leave it open! Schedule no chores or errands; resist organizing the garage. Sometimes you have to give yourself permission to do nothing and be mindless.
- Make these nonnegotiable events just like the other appointments in your day.
- Take a day off work and schedule an appointment at a day spa; plan to spend the entire day there. Doing it on a Friday would be a great choice. Get a full-body massage, herbal wrap, facial, manicure, and pedicure. Have someone drive you home so you can retain your level of relaxation.

▲ ▲ ▲

▼ ▼ ▼

▼ ENERGY BANDIT #4 | **Thinking about work or kids while you relax**

Children also make it difficult to relax. We feel guilty when we don't spend enough time with them; we feel guilty when we lose our cool and yell at them. Let's face it—if children came with "off" switches, we'd all be better parents! During temper tantrums, we could turn them off, gather our composure, and mastermind a creative and patient solution! Parents need to have space from their children on a regular basis, without feeling guilty. You should get away with your spouse (or alone) without the children, whether it's for one evening or one week.

▲ ENERGY BOOSTER | **Don't feel guilty when you play**

Be present in your play and enjoy yourself, without thinking about that unfinished report or the shoes your daughter wants you to buy her. Playing—when you think you should be doing something more productive—might be uncomfortable at first. But if you wait until all your work is done before you play, you will never play. I know of a woman who took a weeklong vacation with her husband; it was the first time in eighteen years they had taken a vacation together without the three kids. They were also caring for her elderly parents. Her sister came for an extended visit, and chased them out of the house so she could look after their kids and the elderly parents. The woman later confided to a friend that she felt guilty leaving the kids with her sister. Her friend said, "Guilty? Are you nuts? You take care of three kids and your ill parents 24–7, 365 days a year! And you feel *guilty* for a taking a week away with your husband?" It was the first time they had the opportunity to be intimate and truly enjoy each other's company in many months.

▲ ▲ ▲
▼ ▼ ▼

▼ ENERGY BANDIT #5 | **Workaholism**

I run into many people who claim they work twelve hours a day because they love their jobs. So what? I have passion for my work too, and you don't find me working that long. This is workaholism, pure and simple. Workaholism, or compulsive work syndrome, is defined as "a compulsive and unrelenting need to work." This term was coined in the 1970s; it is a cousin to obsessive compulsive disorder. Workaholics believe their world will collapse if they don't work. A workaholic doesn't always necessarily love her work or try to excel, but she typically believes she is *the only person capable of performing her work.* This disorder can affect any job, from corporate executive to stay-at-home mom. If you're a workaholic, you should seek counseling.

Working too much and relaxing too little will literally make you sick. Dr. Bryan Robinson, a therapist and professor at the University of North Carolina, says workaholism can lead to headaches, fatigue, depression, high blood pressure, and heart disease. Researchers from the University of Massachusetts Medical School in Shrewsbury tracked more than ten thousand workers and found that working twelve-hour days (no matter what the total work hours were per week) increased risk of injury or illness by 37 percent. A study in the *American Journal of Family Therapy* followed one thousand married couples with one spouse diagnosed as a workaholic; it showed that these couples experienced a 40 percent higher divorce rate than nonworkaholic couples.

▲ ENERGY BOOSTER | **Get help for workaholism**

To recover from workaholism, you have to challenge the social acceptance—even society's encouragement—of these common phrases: "Look how productive you're being. You are accomplishing great things"; "You possess that strong work ethic your father instilled in you. Hard work is good for you." Or perhaps your own self-talk is the problem: "You just love your work—it is your hobby, in fact—you're having so much fun that it just doesn't feel like you're working." The rationalizations abound. Is there incongruence in these words or simply denial?

I am severely unimpressed by people who brag about the long hours they put in each week. It says to me that they are not managing their time well. You have to figure out how to get the results your job requires but do it in less time, leave the office earlier, and get home to a life. If you're working too many hours, perhaps you're not delegating properly. Or you haven't hired enough people. Or you don't trust your assistant. Or you're a perfectionist. Don't get me wrong. It's perfectly normal to work long hours when first starting up a company, for example. It's perfectly normal to occasionally work an eighty-hour week when you have an important project deadline. Then things should go back to normal. But if that becomes a habit, you have a problem.

Start by admitting you have a problem and join a local chapter of Workaholics Anonymous. WA is "a fellowship of individuals who share their experience, strength, and hope with each other that they may solve their common problems and recover from workaholism." To find a support group in your area, go to www.workaholics-anonymous.org or write to P.O. Box 289, Menlo Park, CA 94026–0289, or call 510–273–9253.

▲　▲　▲

▼ ▼ ▼

▼ ENERGY BANDIT #6 | **Being wound up from a stressful day and unable to relax**

You might find it hard to calm down and make a relaxing transition to bedtime. You know how sometimes your to-do list unexpectedly sounds like a giant gong when you're dead asleep, and then your mind starts going 90 mph?

▲ ENERGY BOOSTER | **Try progressive relaxation for thirty minutes**

This will help you get to sleep if you experience insomnia. It also quiets your mind and allows you to get to sleep. Lie on your back, and let your toes gently fall outward to the sides. Place a pillow under your knees if that makes your lower back more comfortable. Let your arms lie along your sides, palms up. This is called the relaxation pose in yoga. Let your thoughts subside. Let your entire body completely relax; if you feel any areas with tension, allow them to loosen. The idea is to go completely limp. Now focus your mind on each body part, starting with your toes, then your feet, then your lower legs, then your knees, and so forth, working your way upward. As you mentally focus on each body part, relax all muscles in that part. Work progressively up through the crown of your head. You can even say a little meditation for each body part: "Thank you, feet, for carrying me wherever I need to go." This also helps bring love and therefore health to each area of your body.[1] The repetitive nature of the meditation focuses yet bores your mind, which is a particularly effective relaxation technique! Your mind will naturally shift to a meditative state, and your brain will begin emitting relaxing alpha waves. Listen to soothing music if you like.

▲ ▲ ▲

▼ ▼ ▼

▼ ENERGY BANDIT #7 | **Not taking all your allotted vacation and personal time each year**

According to the National Institute for Occupational Safety and Health, the primary function of a vacation is to ease stress—some early signs of which include headaches, a short temper, trouble sleeping, and low morale. All of these can have an effect on job performance. According to a survey by Vault, an online career services company, 81 percent of employers and 47 percent of employees have done work while on vacation. Relaxation is not optional; it's a necessity—and can actually improve performance back at work. Studies also show that employees exhibit higher productivity when they take regular vacations and enjoy a healthy balance between work and home life.[2]

Studies have also found that job performance improves after a vacation. Joe Robinson reported a story in the August 13, 2006, *Los Angeles Times* about the H Group, an investment services company in Salem, Oregon, that doubled its income after owner Ron Kelemen increased employee time off to three and a half weeks a year. Robinson also cited a Cincinnati cleaning company, Jancoa, that experienced soaring employee productivity—high enough to cut overtime—after it switched to a three-week vacation policy.

▲ ENERGY BOOSTER | **Take regular vacations**

Human beings need breaks on a larger scale, interjecting regular vacations into their work lives. Stress and leisure are inversely proportional: the less leisure time you build into your overall life, the more stress you will experience. And high stress levels are a recipe for low energy. We all need healthy doses of escaping the soul-hardening world of technology and immersing ourselves in the profound healing power of nature. There's a reason why geographic locations with stunning scenery are popular vacation destinations. Hence the word *recreation*. We re-create, restore, and renew ourselves when we get away from the day-to-day for large periods of time, several times a year.

In order to switch your focus from results to relaxation, you have to be gone long enough to stop thinking about *doing* and shift to *being*. How long should you take? One week can seem too short. Just as you're relaxing, it's time to leave. But two weeks can seem too long, especially if you have your children with you. So I've come to enjoy a compromise at ten days. It's long enough where I can relax and forget what day it is but short enough where I don't come back to an overwhelming workload. If you take these ten days tagged onto Memorial Day weekend, July 4 weekend, or Labor Day weekend, you end up with two full weeks and three weekends, which gives you time at the end of your vacation to get organized and back into the swing of things before work begins. If nothing else, take a long weekend. Go camping, rent a cabin, make reservations at a spa resort—whatever it is that you would love to do. Be cautious about making it a weekend in the big city unless you're really into that; the idea is relaxation, not overstimulation. The goal is peace and quiet.

Part of what makes a vacation restful is getting away from your routine. This can be tricky for people who live in beautiful vacation areas. For example, if you live on a lake, you may not feel a need to "get away." After all, you have a beautiful view of a lake right outside your window. You have to step outside of your life for perspective. You have to get out of your daily routine and your normal environment several times a year—even if it means getting away only for a weekend.

▲ ▲ ▲

▼ ▼ ▼

▼ ENERGY BANDIT #8 | Jamming up your vacation with work

Vacations are not supposed to be productive. Don't try to visit every single site in the vicinity, checking them off like tasks on a to-do list. A vacation isn't about productivity; it's about relaxation. The quality of a vacation isn't measured by the output. How do you quantify fun, play, adventure, rest, and quiet? How do you tally the spray of an exploding waterfall in Kauai? You need to be in a place where all the home-improvement projects and bills aren't staring you in the face. Somewhere where you can step off the hamster wheel of daily drudgery. No schedule, no projects—just big, wide-open spaces of being.

▲ ENERGY BOOSTER | Leave your electronic devices behind when you vacation

Human beings are living organisms, and they need regular infusions of the completely natural, nonsynthetic technological world—not just for a few weeks a year, but on a daily basis too. So when you go on vacation, leave your laptop and BlackBerry *at home*! I know of one man who took his BlackBerry with him on vacation. His extended family members told him they were going to confiscate it if he didn't turn it off and enjoy spending time with them at the lakeshore! Take your cell phone only for emergency purposes. Politely inform your coworkers that you are to be contacted only in the event of an emergency—in other words, if the office burns down. If someone from the office is rude enough to leave a message on your cell phone while you're on vacation, don't even listen to it. When you're on your deathbed, you're not going to wish you had spent more time at the office.

▲ ▲ ▲

Ten

Attitude

I have people in my life I love being around: they lift my spirits and give me joy. Other people just suck the life right out of me: they are so negative, I walk away feeling emotionally drained. Meetings with these "de-energizers" are often unavoidable, so we waste time dreading them and mentally rehearsing how we will cope. After a disheartening interaction, we seek out colleagues to vent our frustrations to, who in turn may experience decreased energy. Thus, negative people not only drain the people they meet but often affect the energy of people they might not even know. Attitude, whether positive or negative, is contagious—what type are you spreading? Being negative really takes extra energy—energy you could otherwise be channeling into your favorite pursuits. This chapter deals with your attitude: the way you look at potentially negative events, your emotional control, the way you perceive people, and your mental perceptions and interpretations of stressful situations. You'll learn how to cultivate tolerance instead of impatience, optimism rather than pessimism, and gratitude over an ungrateful spirit.

▼ ▼ ▼

| **Stinking thinking**

Pessimism, self-doubt, complaining, whining, and general negativity—
it's all the same thing: stinking thinking. Have you ever been around
people who have it made, yet all they do is complain? The movie *Lost
in Translation* is a good example of this. It's basically about well-off people who are miserable all the time. If you're reading this book, chances
are you have a roof over your head, plenty to eat, a reliable vehicle, and
clothes in your closet that you haven't worn in a year. This is not to
equate materialism with happiness, but so many people overlook all
that they have to be grateful for and complain about every tiny little
everyday thing that goes wrong. The milk spills, the faucet starts drip-
ping, the computer crashes. That's just life. Hence the saying "If it's not
one thing, it's another!" The things that go right during the course of
a given day far outweigh the things that go wrong.

▲ ENERGY BOOSTER | **Stop negative thoughts in their tracks**

It's all too easy for us to internalize the harsh messages society feeds
us. Perhaps we endured hypercritical parents or teachers during
childhood. Perhaps we have attended religious institutions that ingrained guilt and shame due to the belief that people are inherently
bad. Perhaps we're constantly bombarded with images of digitally
enhanced supermodels. Monitor your thoughts. Are your thoughts
mostly positive, or mostly negative? Perhaps that's one of the biggest
tests of life—learning how to transform the negative to positive.
Like turning vegetable scraps into rich compost for your daisy garden. Remember the old ditty:

> As you go through life, brother,
> Whatever be your goal,

Keep your eye upon the doughnut,
And not upon the hole!

Would you ever talk to a friend the way you sometimes talk to yourself? Try reassuring yourself the same way you'd reassure a friend. Let's say you're getting ready for work, and you know that your boss is conducting your annual evaluation today, so you're a little nervous. While you're combing your hair, your concerns morph into a little movie inside your head wherein the boss calls you an idiot, you jump to your feet, and a screaming match ensues. Stop that thought immediately! Now replace it with images of your boss giving you ample positive feedback, a great overall evaluation, big smiles on both your faces—and you even get a raise!

Instead of thinking "The board will never put me in the CEO seat because I'm a woman," think "The board is going to name me CEO because I masterminded netting $8.7 million for this company last year!"

Instead of thinking "The bank won't give me that business startup loan because I'm of African descent," think "The loan officer is going to fall all over herself giving me a business startup loan because of my golden credit rating!"

Instead of thinking "They won't hire me, since I'm already fifty-nine," think "They'll hire me in a heartbeat, because I'm a walking encyclopedia of expertise!"

▲ ▲ ▲
▼ ▼ ▼

▼ ENERGY BANDIT #2 | Worrying about everything

Worrying is one of the most ineffective, counterproductive things you can do with the human mind. When you worry, you may be picturing a negative event. In other words, you're creating the exact thing you want to avoid.

▲ ENERGY BOOSTER | Create alternative mental pictures

When you become a parent, your number one concern in life is keeping your children safe and sound. A mother of four young children confided one of her fears to me. At the time, she lived in the valley of a mountainous area that was prone to flash flooding in the spring. She relayed to me that she had a paralyzing fear of a flash flood engulfing her minivan with all four children inside—three of whom still required car seats. How would she alone be able to get all of the smallest three children out of their car seats? And hold them in her arms while swimming? Would the oldest child be a strong enough swimmer to save himself—plus one of the other children? Imagination is a built-in survival tool that has furthered the human race's evolution. But it can rage out of control if you don't keep it in check. This mother's concern was very practical, but it even kept her from wanting to drive in the rain. Yes, you need to have a game plan for emergency situations. But you can't let them consume your mental energy. If you find yourself worrying about a particular scenario, stop thinking about it right away. Then immediately replace it with a positive thought about the same scenario. I told the mother to come up with a game plan and replace her worry with an image of her family always traveling safely on dry roads.

▼ ENERGY BANDIT #3 | Feeling angry all the time

Like worry, anger is an evolutionary tool that keeps us safe. It is very helpful when it comes to protecting ourselves and our loved ones from harm. But if we are chronically angry—internally or outwardly—we are compromising our own health and well-being. The physiological effects of anger involve a two-phase blast of adrenaline-related neurotransmitters called catecholamines. The first blast is a fight-or-flight response to energize the body for immediate action, which lasts for just a few minutes. The second surge persists for as long as several hours to several days. Chronic anger-control problems can predispose us toward cardiac risk factors such as high blood pressure, high cholesterol, and weight gain. These risk factors can trigger a life-threatening heart attack or another coronary event—especially during an explosive outburst. Anger's bad-attitude cousins are frustration, jealousy, resentment, hatred, judgment, and criticism.

▲ ENERGY BOOSTER | **Listen to what your anger is teaching you**

Because anger is a normal human emotion, you have to respond to it carefully. Even the calmest of personalities erupts in anger now and then. It requires a great deal of restraint on our part to rationally deal with others when they are explosively angry—and to properly channel and express our own anger. Instead of lashing out, become introspective about what it's trying to tell you. Perhaps you are discovering boundaries that need to be set with another person. Perhaps it will teach you how to deal more effectively with a difficult personality. As you learn these lessons and put them into action, your behavior will naturally create maximum pressure for other people to act fairly toward you. If you're faced with someone who's explosively angry, remain calm. Of course, this is harder than it sounds. But throwing an entire container of lighter fluid on the already raging fire is never a good idea. Breathe deeply and slowly. Use a calm tone of voice; politely explain that there's no need to yell, and that you're open to listening to his or her concerns.

▲ ▲ ▲

▼ ▼ ▼

▼ ENERGY BANDIT #4 | Dealing with emotionally charged situations

A host of a children's television program in the Midwest in the 1970s, Cowboy Bob, closed every show by saying, "If you can't say anything nice, don't say anything at all!" If only more adults abided by this simple philosophy, the world would be a much nicer place. Some people are otherwise intelligent, but they have a brusque communication style. Some people could receive a silver platter stacked with $1 million, and they would ask irritably, "Where's the whipped cream with the cherry on top?" Some people rub you the wrong way no matter what, and you can't quite put your finger on it. Simply being around them makes you tired.

▲ ENERGY BOOSTER | Douse the flames of emotionally charged situations

Sometimes you simply have to adjust your own attitude to deal effectively with others' personality quirks:

- Don't interrupt when someone is venting; listen to the other person, no matter how illogical his or her words are. And don't let the other person interrupt you; politely ask to be listened to.
- If necessary, state, "If you are so upset that you are unable to exercise basic courtesy and allow me to finish my sentences, perhaps we should cool off for a bit before we continue this discussion." Cooling off may take five minutes, five hours, or five days.
- Don't allow the other person to become verbally abusive. If the other person calls you names, refuse to continue the con-

versation. "I refuse to listen to anyone who treats me with disrespect. We can continue this discussion after you've calmed down." Physically remove yourself from the situation.

- If you have to be around someone who is chronically toxic—is verbally abusive and has anger-control problems—consider permanently removing yourself from the situation. If your boss makes your stomach hurt, consider changing jobs. Sometimes we can adapt our attitude to interact productively with such personalities. But you have to know where to draw the line to protect your own well-being and up your chronically low energy and motivation levels.

▲ ▲ ▲
▼ ▼ ▼

▼ ENERGY BANDIT #5 | Being a pessimist

Are you the kind of person who gets an ulcer from receiving an A- instead of an A+? Do you always focus on what you don't have instead of what you do have? Do all the little things that go wrong during the course of an average day make you think the universe is out to get you? Optimists and pessimists view the exact same thing from entirely different viewpoints. This reminds me of a little joke I heard: The optimist falls down on his front porch and breaks his arm. He says, "Gee whiz! I'm glad that happened to me and not to someone else!" The pessimist says to him, "Are you some kind of masochistic nutcase?" The optimist replies, "Of course not! But if it had been someone else, I might get sued!" The optimist realizes that no matter how bad something is, it could always be worse.

▲ ENERGY BOOSTER | Choose to be an optimist today

If you really think about it, happiness is a *choice*. That's assuming all your basic needs are met, of course. If life throws lemons at you, make lemonade. Pessimists forget to laugh. Optimists laugh to forget. Keep it in perspective. Remember, things can always be worse. Be grateful for what you *do* have. So three things went wrong during your morning—big deal! Think of all the countless things that went *right*: you had enough hot water to take a shower, the car started, and you arrived at the office safely. Having a bad attitude about a particular circumstance will not make that circumstance go away. But having a bad attitude will drain your energy and make an already bad situation even worse. Focus on the positive, not the negative. So the unexpected furnace repair is going to cost four hundred dollars? Be glad you have more than four hundred dollars in your checking account. Having a positive attitude helps take the sting out of an unexpected occurrence and boosts your energy to deal with it.

▼ ENERGY BANDIT #6 | An ungrateful spirit

I love sitting in first class on an airplane. By policy, I travel coach to my speaking engagements. Occasionally, I will earn enough upgrade certificates in my mileage program to upgrade myself to first class, even though I'm paying only for a coach ticket. I feel blessed each time I get to sit there and would expect others to feel the same way. But once I had a seatmate who complained about *everything*—the seats, the food, and the lack of choices on the menu. Excuse me? A lack of choices? The people in coach are jealous that we even have food! And this guy's complaining about sitting in first class. Are you that way? Do you complain in first class?

▲ ENERGY BOOSTER | Count your blessings

Stop complaining about what you don't have and start counting up all the things you do have! I give training seminars at an accounting firm in Denver, Colorado, that has been awarded the "Best Place to Work in Denver" three years in a row. After the busy tax season has ended, the partners of the firm regularly hand out goodies: extra days of vacation, a one-hundred-dollar gift card, or a video iPod. Every time I'm there to teach, the firm orders food for the class participants, and there are free sodas, coffee, and tea every day. Unbelievably, one woman in my seminar was complaining about the company not providing energy drinks. I couldn't believe my ears! I told her she had absolutely no idea how spoiled she was and she should count her blessings.

Counting your blessings is an instant energy boost. At the University of California at Riverside, psychologist Sonja Lyubomirsky used grant money from the National Institutes of Health to study different kinds of happiness boosters. One tool was the gratitude journal, a diary in which subjects write down things for which they are thankful. Lyubomirsky found that conscientiously counting your blessings once a week will significantly increase your overall satisfaction with life over a period of six weeks, whereas a control group that did not keep journals had no such gain.[1] At the University of California at Davis, psychologist Robert Emmons found that people who keep gratitude journals improve physical health, raise energy levels, and report fewer physical symptoms. "The ones who benefited most tended to elaborate more and have a wider span of things they're grateful for," he noted. So get out a piece of paper and write down all the wonderful things in your life.

▲ ▲ ▲

▼ ▼ ▼

Intolerance of others

If only everyone would do what they're supposed to do when they're supposed to do it, and do a good job, life would be so much simpler. It is common for high-functioning, intelligent people to become impatient or frustrated with others. It's also easy for people with a particular type of intelligence to become frustrated with others who don't excel in that area. Some people may be capable of writing a Pulitzer Prize–winning book, but are completely stumped when it comes to screwing in a lightbulb.

▲ ENERGY BOOSTER | **Cultivate patience with people**

From personality quirks to learning styles, others' differences can sour our attitude, draining our energy. By cultivating patience toward other people's forms of intelligence and learning styles, and transforming any subtle prejudices we may harbor, we can lighten the load of dealing with others. Here are some ideas to help you relate to other people:

- If you dislike someone, force yourself to find one thing, just one—I know it's hard—that you like about him or her. This will help give you the stamina to continue working with that person.
- Recognize that different people have different learning styles. Some people need to have a ten-minute meeting to bounce ideas off others aloud. Some people can't follow oral instructions—they have to be written. Some people have problems with reading comprehension. Some people can't synthesize what's covered in a presentation at a conference unless they take copious notes. Be sure to recognize your own, and oth-

ers', learning styles. Request to receive information in a format that is easy for you to assimilate; likewise, provide information to others in a format that is easy for them to assimilate.

- Double-check your belief system. Don't subconsciously stereotype others' abilities based on gender, race, age, background, and so forth.
- Double-check any rigidity and perfectionism you may be exhibiting. It doesn't matter *how* someone performs at a task, as long as it's accomplished within the required time frame and meets your quality standards.
- If others' personality quirks annoy you at an infrequent event—such as getting together with family during the holidays—then pretend you're in a sitcom or novel teeming with eccentric personalities. Sit back and let yourself be entertained!
- Do something unexpected. You regularly avoid Susie-Q because she is negative. Invite her to lunch. Really listen.
- Realize that you too are not perfect. Learn to laugh at your own foibles, and you'll naturally develop more patience when others make mistakes.

▲ ▲ ▲
▼ ▼ ▼

▼ ENERGY BANDIT #8 | **Playing psychoanalyst to the people who annoy you**

If someone puts barbs into your skin, it's most likely about him or her, not about you. Maybe he had an argument with his spouse that morning. Maybe she had a flat tire on the way to work. Sometimes people just have a bad day, and they're grumpy, and it has nothing to do with you.

▲ ENERGY BOOSTER | **Don't waste your time overanalyzing people**

There's not always an ulterior motive behind what people do. Don't take someone else's bad mood personally. Sometimes a spade is just a spade. Don't read too much into what people say. You can even take a second to cheer up a grumpy person. Send an e-card. Share a special treat you planned to eat yourself. It takes only a few seconds to be nice. Happiness is contagious. But of course if the barbs are chronic, you should politely bring his or her attention to it. Or consider minimizing or eliminating your contact with that person if necessary.

▲ ▲ ▲

Eleven

Resolution

Isn't it amazing how much energy you can spend stewing about things? When I'm irritated or frustrated, I can *feel* my energy flowing out. When my computer is causing problems, I get so agitated, I'm completely unable to focus on any other task. Until I can calmly address the issue, I'm no good.

The last chapter talked about mental energy. This chapter discusses how to create closure on the things in your life that bother you: you are going to *do* something about them. What are you tolerating? When do you experience frustration? What do you do when someone wastes your time? All of those situations require closure, so that you can direct your energy to more positive pursuits. Some frustrations you can fix—like a computer or a watch in need of a new battery. Others you can't eliminate—like relatives—but you can communicate how their actions affect you. Perhaps your coworker is constantly gossiping and trying to suck you into her problems. You'll create boundaries for yourself that don't come across as uncaring to others. We'll work on those little problems and open loops nagging at your mind, to free it up for energy expenditure on more worthwhile endeavors.

▼ ▼ ▼

▼ ENERGY BANDIT #1 | **Dealing with energy vampires**

Okay, let's face it: humans are the most annoying species on the planet. They're the source of all that's wrong with the world, after all: poverty, war, global warming, you name it. The elephants and monkeys are just minding their own business eating leaves and fruit from the trees, but those humans! Ugh!

I read a fascinating study in the *Journal of Personality and Social Psychology* that researched what would happen to your ability to concentrate on a task (such as writing) after you're forced to work with another person or coordinate a task (such as cooking). The results showed that when the effort with the other person was perceived as efficient and effortless (low-maintenance), the individual had no trouble working on subsequent, unrelated tasks. However, when the interaction with the individual was high-maintenance—inefficient, effortful, and frustrating—subjects were unfocused and unmotivated when trying to work on an unrelated task later that day. In other words, working with a high-maintenance individual can sap your energy so much that it renders you unable to concentrate and the quality of your work declines. No wonder we complain about having to work with certain people—they can ruin us for the day![1]

▲ ENERGY BOOSTER | **Avoid energy vampires**

You know who they are: the people in your life who drain your energy in five minutes flat. They may be beautiful on the outside, but they are ugly on the inside. These are the most common types:

- People who criticize you constantly. This includes coworkers, "friends," and even extended family members and your parents. Spend as little time as possible around these people and choose to end relationships with friends who take and take and never give back. If it's a relative, set specific boundaries about when, where, and how often you'll get together.

- People who constantly whine, complain, and kvetch. This reminds me of a T-shirt I saw in a catalog: "I had a nice day, and I didn't like it!" These people have it made, but if one pebble gets into their shoe, they'll whine about how it ruined their entire week. Find other people to hang out with who don't ruin your good mood.

- People who gossip or try to create drama. Perhaps it's someone in your extended family who's retired and bored, or the queen of gossip at the office. These people are always trying to sweep you up in a web of interpersonal turmoil.

- People who are just plain rude. Maybe they're chauvinists, maybe they're overcompensating for having a fragile ego—who cares what the reason is. Avoid them. Don't do what you may have done in high school—following them around, trying to get them to like you. Maybe they're otherwise great people, care about the same social issues you do, are very creative, but they're just plain rude, mean, obnoxious, brusque, and abrasive. They dig hurtful barbs into your very being with their mean words. Life's too short to hang around these people.

- Mean people. Does someone hate you for no good reason you can think of? I know of a woman who has a stepmother who flat-out said to her the very first time she met her: "Everyone in the family has told me about how pretty and smart you are. Well, I don't believe that anyone is that good. I decided before I ever met you that I didn't like you." Needless to say, she steers a very wide berth around her "stepmonster."

▲ ▲ ▲

▼ ▼ ▼

▼ ENERGY BANDIT #2 | Not stating your needs

No matter how annoying other people are, sometimes we're afraid that if we clearly communicate our needs, we'll hurt their feelings. Maybe we're trying to be good Christians or Buddhists or spouses or parents or coworkers. But don't confuse repression with politeness; it's completely possible, even advisable, to communicate your needs in a polite and sensitive manner.

▲ ENERGY BOOSTER | Practice preventive assertions with annoying situations

As the old saying goes, "An ounce of prevention is worth a pound of cure!" Be assertive. But being assertive is *not* the same as being aggressive. Being assertive simply means that you express your feelings and needs in a polite manner. And no, you don't have to engage in some long, drawn-out discussion. You don't have to hold a UN peace conference; it takes only a few minutes to communicate clearly.

Does your husband leave his clean laundry on the dresser instead of putting it away? Don't let it fester; it will morph into resentment inside you, which will eventually affect your relationship. Instead of biting your lip because you know he's been swamped at work, you need to politely say, "If you could please put away your laundry on laundry day, it would be a big help for my stress level." Or if dirty clothes are strewn all over the floor, you could say, "One of my responsibilities is the laundry, and I will be happy to wash whatever clothes are in the hamper." Your teenager leaves her homework papers and books all over the couch? Don't stifle yourself because you know she's stressed out about homework. Just politely state, "You need to get all your stuff out of the living room before bedtime."

You could likewise ask your family members or your coworkers if there's anything *you* could change in your own behavior that would help them. This can even be a funny topic of conversation at the dinner table. One woman and her teenager were enjoying dinner together; the teenager was complaining about some of her father's annoying habits. So the mother asked, "What about me drives you nuts?" The teenager seemed hesitant to reply, but the mother grinned and said, "*Everybody* has annoying habits! What are some of mine?" The teenager calmly relayed to her mother that she talked really loud on the phone, and that she explained instructions for doing things around the house as if she were talking to a little kid. So now when the mother catches herself doing these things, she stops—and winks at her teenager. One boss was conducting an annual evaluation of one of his employees. When the evaluation was finished, he asked, "Now, what can *I* do to make things easier for *you*?" His employee thought this was particularly generous and practical, not to mention a big relief. It gave her a chance to tell him that instead of giving her creative leeway on a project then wanting her to overhaul it later because he had something else in mind, it would save them both a lot of time and effort if he would communicate his suggestions and desires at the outset.

▲ ▲ ▲
▼ ▼ ▼

▼ ENERGY BANDIT #3 | Tasks that you want to do "someday" that aren't urgent

There may be certain items on your to-do list that seem to hover there for all eternity due to perceived lack of time. These things range from home-improvement projects to making vacation travel plans to repairing broken items. They might be things that take more time than you can accomplish on a weeknight, but that you don't want to waste your weekend time doing. These things are like small children tugging at your skirts; they're *not* going to stop annoying you until you tend to them.

▲ ENERGY BOOSTER | **Set aside a day to clear up nagging mental reminders**

- Find those couple of things on your to-do list that have been staring you in the face for longer than two months. Do them. Make that list of phone calls. Clear all the scrawled notes to yourself from the telephone table.

- Take those envelopes of photographs and sort them into photo boxes by month. Take them out of the packages, file them behind index cards, and write the events on the front of each card.

- Fix it if it's broken. Has your "check engine" light been on for two months, but you "don't have time" to take it to the auto mechanic? Is that chipped paint on the kitchen wall driving you buggy? The shutter's been jammed on your 35-mm camera for an entire year, and you've been forcing yourself to use a digital camera that you hate? Not only do broken things dam up in your mind and sap your energy, but they also make you feel impoverished. If the hubcap on your car is missing, replace it. Just do it. Yes, you do have the time and money. You're not going to miss a deadline or go broke if you accomplish these trivial tasks that have been pecking at you for months on end.

- Dive into those piles of paper that are multiplying like bunnies on your desk. Force yourself to do one of six Ds:
  1. Discard (toss or recycle)
  2. Delegate (route to someone else)
  3. Do (immediately)
  4. Date (file in a tickler/suspense file)

5. Drawer (file in your reference files)

6. Deter (get yourself removed from the distribution list)

▲ ▲ ▲
▼ ▼ ▼

Many of us are continually frustrated by the number of "half-done" things in our lives. You plan for a big business trip, get the travel arranged, make hotel reservations, register for the conference—and it goes off without a hitch. Now you have a pile of receipts that sit there for a month and stare at you. You didn't complete the trip, because you still need to write up the expense report and close out the file. This type of incompletion will drain your energy and frustrate you every time you look at it.

You could have twenty to fifty half-done tasks sitting around your office and home. You read a great article in a magazine and thought, "I should send that to Mom." You bookmarked the page, closed the magazine, put it on your coffee table—and pass it ten times a day, each time saying to yourself, "I should send that article to Mom." Your daughter is studying French at school, and you'd love to be able to converse with her and possibly visit France together someday. So you purchase these nifty "Teach Yourself French" tapes . . . and you never take them out of the box.

Nagging reminders of postponed tasks will leave you frustrated. Finishing things and moving them through to full completion will have a dramatic impact on your energy and enthusiasm. Sometimes it feels like you have a lot more to do than in actuality, because you have lots of small details weighing on your mind. Here are some ways to gain closure:

- Unpack and reorganize as soon as you return from a trip, processing all information through your system and getting it into the right place.
- Invoice your client or company immediately following each job or business trip, so that you keep receipts in order and get every dime you're entitled to receive.
- Label videotapes immediately after running out of tape, indicating the contents on the cover, and filing with the rest.
- After pulling artwork out of your child's backpack, toss the nonoriginal items. Immediately write a date on the back of the ones you want to save, and put them in a drawer or plastic bin of that child's treasures.
- Return a book you borrowed from a friend and completed months ago but never gave back due to embarrassment. Put it in your car in a bag, leave it on that person's front porch, and e-mail him or her saying, "I was in your area and didn't call first, so I didn't want to bother you, but I left your book on the porch. Can we set up a lunch date?" You cleared up the issue that was bothering you and paved the way to connect again.
- Enter information from business cards you receive after conferences into your database or contact-management software. Follow up.

Get in the habit of doing things from beginning to end; move things through the system from start to finish. Resolve to stop doing things halfway. Stop thinking about doing it. Like the Nike commercial says: Just do it!

▲ ▲ ▲

▼ ▼ ▼

▼ ENERGY BANDIT #5 | Wasting time waiting

It's bad enough when we waste time, but it's even worse when someone wastes it for us. For example, people always tell me how lucky I am to have the opportunity to be on television. "Wow, it must be nice to be such a celebrity!" they say. I was scheduled to appear on a national television show on June 26, 2006, to be interviewed live about my newest book, *Find More Time*. I give up a weekend with my family and make the long trek from Denver to New York City on Sunday. I arrive, fight New York City traffic for ninety minutes, check into my hotel, get something to eat alone (by the way, Sarabeth's Kitchen—www.sarabeth.com—has the best tomato soup I've ever had; their preserves are fabulous too), and sit down to think about the interview. The phone rings. It's the PR rep for my publisher. "Your segment's been bumped," she says. "Huh?" I ask, intelligently. "Oh, don't worry; they're still going to tape it." I flew all the way to New York for a live interview that will now be a taped interview, which I could have done in the CBS studio twenty minutes up the road from me. I had just sent an e-mail out to my list of ten thousand subscribers to watch the show. "That's just the way television is," everyone reassured me. Maybe they need to hire me to teach them a time-management lesson.

▲ ENERGY BOOSTER | Occupy yourself productively while waiting

Like my television experience, you can't always do something about it when others waste your time and force you to wait. (Security lines in the airport also come to mind.) When a potential client of yours is late for a meeting, and you're waiting alone in the lobby or restaurant, you could certainly leave. But then you would waste all the time it took you to get there, you'd have to reschedule, and you'd potentially lose the business. So instead, plan ahead in the *event* that you'll have to wait for someone, so that you don't get agitated and can be productive. By assuming you'll have to wait, you'll have something to do should that happen, and not end up frustrated. If you plan to show up early for your flight, you can be productive in the gate area, rather than plopping down, exhausted, in your plane seat, seconds away from missing your plane. If the cable guy is going to need a four-hour window for an appointment, what can you accomplish while waiting, rather than sitting there watching TV?

Here are some things you can do while waiting:

- Catch up on your reading.
- Pay bills.
- Write a few thank-you notes.
- Sort mail.
- File while on hold (wear a wireless headset).
- Answer e-mail on your handheld.
- Stroll around the soccer field while waiting for your kid to finish up practice.
- Make some phone calls (use Bluetooth so you can talk and walk at the same time if necessary).
- Write out a grocery list.
- Plan your next month.
- Call your mother.

▼ ENERGY BANDIT #6 | **Boredom**

You crawl out of bed, put your feet on the floor, and groan, "Oh, God, it's Monday." Wouldn't you rather feel like "Hooray! Thank God it's Monday!"? Does your daily life resemble the movie *Ground-*

hog Day? Are you doing the same things every day? Wake up, get ready for work, fight traffic, work like crazy, fight traffic, fix dinner as close to the speed of light as possible, drive kid number 1 to soccer practice number 1, drive kid number 2 to swimming practice number 2, drive home, supervise homework and bath time, do dishes and chores, go to bed, get up and do it all over again. This reminds me of a punk song from the eighties by The Godfathers: "Birth, School, Work, Death!"

▲ ENERGY BOOSTER | **Mix it up a little**

Maybe you're intellectually unfulfilled. Maybe you're spiritually unfulfilled. Maybe you're just tired of the same old daily grind. You need to get out of that rut with some new activities that will be a shot in the arm and stave off boredom:

- Go hear a free lecture. The calendar section in the back of your city's *Business Journal* lists weekly activities.
- Go to a concert that's not in your preferred genre. If you usually attend symphonies, go to a rock concert. If you usually go to rock concerts, attend a symphony. You might be surprised at what else you like.
- Tune the radio to a station geared toward twenty-somethings. Get out of your NPR, golden-oldies, and classic-rock rut. Some of the songs might make you cringe, but there's bound to be a few in there that you like. Then purchase music by the bands you like. This helps keep you young.
- Get an updated haircut. Sure, that style looks great on you— just like it has for the past fifteen years. An updated haircut will make you look and feel years younger.
- Purchase or check out a book from the library that's at the opposite end of the spectrum from what you normally read. Do you love a good mystery? Read a biography instead.

- Change the order of your morning routine. Do you brush your teeth after you shower? Do it beforehand. Do you wash your face over the sink? Try it in the shower instead. Do you eat breakfast before you exercise? Try eating after you exercise. Just mix up the smallest details of your morning routine a little.

- Alter your route to work. A woman I know was tired of sitting in backed-up traffic every single morning on the way to work. So one day on a whim, she just turned onto a side street. She discovered a meandering suburban road atop a ridge with beautiful views of a river valley below. It turned out to be a shortcut that saved her ten minutes getting to work; this became her preferred route. It was a scenic drive that put her in a good mood, which is a great way to start the day.

- Paint one of your rooms a wild color. I know a woman who painted her kitchen yellow. Not just harmonious yellow, but *screaming* yellow. She readily admits that it's tacky, and that she's perfectly aware of the fact that it's an interior designer's nightmare. She says, "Why wait until you're old to be eccentric? Besides, it makes me happy."

▲ ▲ ▲
▼ ▼ ▼

▼ ENERGY BANDIT #7 | **Feeling generally annoyed and irritable**

You can't quite put your finger on it, but you're gritchy, grumbly, and snarky. Everyone is getting on your last nerve. You're impatient, and you're taking your frustrations out on everyone, from the family dog to the children to the innocent cashier at the grocery store. Maybe it's no one's fault but your own.

▲ ENERGY BOOSTER | Look within for the source of your frustration

Rather than looking to external circumstances, perhaps you need to look within. What's bothering you? What's making you so frustrated? What's the number-one thing in your life that makes you want to burst into tears at any moment? When you're feeling agitated, you can usually pinpoint the source of your woes if you think about it long enough.

Maybe the boss snapped at you; you received an unexpected bill; you're feeling overworked and barely keeping up; or maybe you're feeling unfulfilled. Perhaps you are tolerating people and situations that are subconsciously bothersome—the friend who always manages to get in a little dig about how spoiled you are; the messy room in your home you keep locked when visitors arrive; the coworker who expects you to do his job for him; the car making a funny noise; or your teenager's uncouth behavior and profane language. Sometimes it's technology. I had a printer that was annoying me because it took so long to warm up. I bought a new, faster one, and, as silly as it sounds, I felt like the sun just came up. Decide right now to resolve anything you're tolerating, and watch your energy soar.

▲ ▲ ▲
▼ ▼ ▼

▼ ENERGY BANDIT #8 | An inability to say no

Realize that every time you say yes to one thing, you are saying no to another. There is always a trade-off or opportunity cost. You can't be in two different places or do two different things at once. When you give your energy to one activity, you decrease the amount of energy (and time!) you can give to the other. Every time you say yes to one of the hundreds of daily urgent e-mails and phone calls, you are saying no to more family time. Other people will always try to place deadlines on you. If you don't determine what you need to accomplish and how to spend your time, other people will be happy to do it for you. You will never be given an opportunity to say yes to something important—like getting a degree, going to the health club, or getting away for a vacation—unless you say no to other things. The local university is not going to call you and tell you to sign up for a class. The beach is not going to insist you book a vacation. Your health-club representative is not going to e-mail you and insist that you show up and work out for thirty minutes each day. You are going to have to create the space in your life to say yes to those things. Only you can learn to set boundaries and make time for what's important.

▲ ENERGY BOOSTER | **Set limits and boundaries with others**

Saying no is about setting healthy parameters for yourself and recognizing reality. It is about protecting your energy level, your overall productivity, your sanity, and your health. Accept your limitations and focus on what's most important. When people try to spend too much of your time, you must say no to requests. Saying no is *not* the same as being rude. Saying no is not going to make you a bad parent. Saying no is not going to make you lose your job. Saying no will make others admire your strength, resolve, and common-sense practicality. Saying no is simply about acknowledging reality in a polite manner.

When the boss asks you if you can come in on Saturday to finish the quarterly report, reply with something akin to, "I have prior obligations, but I can definitely have it to you by noon on Monday." The boss doesn't have to know that "obligations" means playing with the kids at the beach. If you're given a new project you can't squeeze into your schedule, say, "I'm overcommitted right now; if I take this on, I'll have to stop work on another project. What would you like me to put aside for now?"

It's similar with family members. "Mom, can you give me a manicure tonight?" "I'll tell you what. Although I can't do that right now, I'll give you a manicure *and* a pedicure Friday night after dinner. Then we can watch a movie of your choice while your nails dry. Does that sound like fun?"

One woman asked me, "I'm an admin, so I'm essentially in a customer-support role, and my job is to give people the information they request. How can I say no to them?" The answer isn't necessarily to say no, but to ask questions. Many times we assume people mean "right now" when they ask for things. Specifically say, "Do you need it today, or will Monday be okay?" Or, "Here's a list of the things I'm working on today. Does this take priority?" Have your boss or customer help you prioritize the order.

▲ ▲ ▲

Twelve

Responsibilities

If I didn't do this, would anybody notice?

Unfortunately, not all of our tasks excite us. We downright dislike some responsibilities, and spending energy on them feels wasteful. If an activity is not a challenge or has no reward in it, motivation is difficult. After a long day at work, do you come home to, well, more work? If you're a stay-at-home parent, you may never seem to stop working. Bill paying, cleaning, shopping, cooking . . . it's a seemingly endless list of responsibilities. Spending energy completing low-value tasks at work feels like a waste of time. Wouldn't it be wonderful if you could complete your tasks more efficiently, so you would have energy to spare?

▼ ▼ ▼

▼ ENERGY BANDIT #1 | **Domestic duties**

The very second you walk through the door you're bombarded with requests about dinner, playtime, and homework assistance, plus the latest domestic details from your spouse. And that's not to mention the day's stack of mail, voice messages, and e-mails. And Jennifer has soccer practice at 6:30, and Jason has a piano recital at 7:30.

Parents lead more harried lives today than in previous generations. In many households, both parents have full-time jobs. The Economic Policy Institute in Washington, D.C., found in a 2001 study that from 1989 to 1998, middle-class parents' work hours increased by 246 hours per year—that's six weeks. Add each child's extracurricular activity schedule to that, and all relaxing family time on evenings and weekends has been replaced with household chores, grocery shopping, and errands.

▲ ENERGY BOOSTER | **Develop an evening routine for all family members**

This begins the *second* you walk through the door. By developing an evening routine, you can retain your sanity, happiness, and energy level, and teach members of your family how to respect others' boundaries. Communicating clearly and politely will help children realize that Mommy and Daddy are people too—with their own needs. You can consider the following evening rituals:

- If you dress up for work, change your clothes. This is the first thing you do, period. Nothing else comes first unless there's blood involved. Throw off your shoes, and slip out of those work clothes and into your lounge pants. Even if you have to leave again that evening, trade your work clothes for more comfortable and casual clothing. Pat a cool washcloth over your face or run moistened cotton swabs under your eyes to refresh yourself. Politely explain to your family that you need these five minutes to yourself so that you'll be better able to help them.
- Assist with and/or check homework, if relevant. Work before play.
- Enjoy playtime with your children. Remember the saying "The best thing you can spend on your children is time." Use playtime as the payoff for completing homework and

domestic-duty time. This might mean playing with toys, shooting hoops, or playing a board game with the entire family. Even teenagers will want to hang out with you regularly, though they would never admit it; their "playtime" might be watching their favorite *Veronica Mars* episode on DVD.

- Set a regular bath time for children. Teenagers may want to shower in the morning since they're more concerned with their appearance, and that's fine. They'll likely have more homework that will take up time in the evening.

- Set a regular bedtime for children. Young children need ten to twelve hours of sleep, and teenagers need at least ten hours of sleep. Between bath time and bedtime is the bedtime routine. This can include the child tidying his or her room, packing the backpack for the next day, and a calming bedtime story. Turn off the TV, dim the lights in the child's room, and minimize stimulation—no tickling, no wrestling, and no jumping on the bed. Even teenagers need a fixed bedtime. They will argue and beg to stay up later. To prove your point, you can conduct an experiment. Let your teenager stay up as late as he or she wants to. After one or two days of this, your adolescent will be sleep-deprived, and probably won't argue about going to bed on time that evening. You won't even have to say "I told you so."

▲ ▲ ▲
▼ ▼ ▼

▼ ENERGY BANDIT #2 | The daily grind of cooking dinner

Can you imagine how much simpler our lives would be if we didn't have to eat? We'd save truckloads of money and decades of time. No meal planning, no grocery shopping, no cooking, no cleanup. But we have to eat to live; there's no way around it.

▲ ENERGY BOOSTER | Enlist help with meals

Meal preparation time and cleanup time will decrease if everyone pitches in. And it will also prevent stress, resentment, and energy drain. To get others to help, try some of these ideas:

- Children must learn to cook. Older children and your spouse can chop vegetables. Children can set the table and get out condiments. Each family member should also assist with cleanup. Everyone can have a specific assignment that rotates from week to week to prevent boredom and dread, such as clearing the table, sweeping the floor, loading the dishwasher, washing any items by hand, and storing leftovers.

- Go to the grocery store the same weeknight every week. Notice that I said "weeknight." Weekends are not for running errands. Weekends are for recreation to recharge your batteries. Besides, the grocery is more crowded on weekends; it will be more stressful and take longer. Figure out which night of the week is least crowded at the grocery. Hint: It's not Friday. Purchase everything you're going to need for a full week. This will reduce multiple trips to the grocery for just a handful of forgotten items, saving you time and energy. You will need ingredients for seven dinners, plus enough items for seven breakfasts and seven lunches for the whole family. Sticking with this number saves you time in the grocery store and streamlines your weekly budget. Know how much it costs you per week, and stick to that budget. Make a list of any ingredients you're likely to forget. Children can accompany you and go on a "scavenger hunt" for items on your list, decreasing your time in the store.

- Cook more than your family will eat; leftovers make the easiest, healthiest, and cheapest lunches. Just put the leftovers into a container, pop it into the fridge, and then put it in your briefcase the next morning. And don't forget the fresh fruits and vegetables to accompany it.

▲ ▲ ▲
▼ ▼ ▼

▼ ENERGY BANDIT #3 | Allowing others to sap your energy

Have you ever noticed how clean the house stays when your spouse and children are gone? Have you ever noticed how much work you get done when your supervisor and coworkers are away? No matter how efficient we are, the habits of others can be giant stop signs smack in the middle of our energy expressway. The boss interrupts your flow with spur-of-the-moment meetings three times a week and countless head-pokes into your office to pile yet another meaningless project onto your already overloaded plate. The family cleaned the house last night, but the kids are still leaving their dirty socks all over the living room. Rather than telling them to put their dirty socks in the laundry hamper, you do it yourself because it's easier than having to ask them more than once or dealing with an argument from them. Our stress builds up, and before we realize it, we're screaming at everyone within a five-mile radius and can't figure out why.

▲ ENERGY BOOSTER | Divvy up chores among family members

Every single member of the family should contribute to household chores, as age allows. Try not to make chores gender-specific. Girls should know how to mow the lawn, and boys should know how to cook. These are basic life skills that they'll need as adults. You'll be doing their future college roommates and spouses a favor, making for happy and healthy households. The worst thing parents can do when it comes to household chores is to do it themselves without teaching children how; this even holds true for stay-at-home parents. If you don't teach your children to chip in equally or even how to perform a certain task, you're setting them up for shock and confusion when they move out of the house. Cleanliness is not about having a home worthy of a *Better Homes and Gardens* magazine feature, it's about basic sanitation and health. Create some ground rules like the following:

- Each member of the family should always clean up his or her own mess, such as after fixing a snack or getting out toys.
- Make a list of all daily household chores: mealtime setup and cleanup, taking out trash and recycling, and pet care. Assign the same number of tasks to everyone in the household. Rotate them so children learn how to perform each task, which also adds variety.
- Make a list of all weekly basic sanitation chores: kitchen, bathrooms, floors, dusting. Rotate them from week to week. There is no law written in stone that the house has to be cleaned all in one evening. With a large family to divide chores among, cleaning the entire house in one evening may be accomplished relatively quickly. But with a smaller family, or with children who have extracurricular activities on different evenings, this may not be the case; simply spread cleaning duties over two or more evenings.
- Laundry: Each member of the family could do one or two loads of his or her own laundry on a given night of the week, or family members could take turns being in charge of laundry day from week to week.
- Lawn care: Like mealtime cleanup, each family member could be assigned a specific task, such as picking up sticks, mowing, pulling weeds, or trimming. These can be rotated from week to week so everyone learns how to perform each task, and to provide variety. In snowy climates in winter,

snow blowing plus shoveling sidewalks, steps, porches, and decks can likewise be assigned.

▲ ▲ ▲
▼ ▼ ▼

▼ ENERGY BANDIT #4 | Lack of dialogue about your preferences

We're all guilty of it. We take on too much, and we don't clearly communicate our needs to others. We're afraid we'll appear weak or inept if we ask for assistance. We don't communicate our preferences regarding the habits of others, afraid we'll come across as rude.

▲ ENERGY BOOSTER | Communicate clearly

Clear communication is vital in the workplace and in the home. Use the following clear communication techniques to save you time and energy.

- Don't assume that you know what someone means when they're assigning you a task. Ask questions. Have them clarify. Sometimes others unintentionally or inadvertently withhold information. Perhaps they're in a hurry; perhaps they know you always understand instructions and do an exceptional job; perhaps they have a subconscious fear that you will get promoted above them. Even if you think you know what someone means, *confirm*. If you proceed without confirming and it turns out they wanted something different, you've lost all that time, and you have to start over. In other words, you've just bunched up your schedule, which adds to your stress level.

- Say "please" and "thank you." People love to be appreciated. When someone accomplishes a task, be sure to thank them: "Thanks so much for cleaning the bathrooms." This is an especially good example for children. Being thanked tells them that they're important. And they respond better to polite requests rather than to yelling. And they definitely respond to enumerated reasons why instead of "Because I told you so." "Jason, could you pick up your toys from the stairs right away, please? I wouldn't want you to trip over one and break your leg. I'd much rather play tag with you than drive you to the emergency room."

- A little humor goes a long way. "You want it *today*? Well, that's too late. I'll give it to you yesterday. But really, I can get it to you by eleven AM tomorrow. Does that work for you?"

- Challenge unrealistic deadlines. We live in a fast-food, instant-messaging, expressway-speeding society, and people want their requests *now*. But now, or even ASAP, isn't possible in this time-space continuum. Perhaps you need to question deadlines when people do the equivalent of asking a gourmet chef to deliver a meal to your table in seven minutes. Having inadequate time to accomplish a task compromises quality. Sometimes unrealistic deadline requests are the symptom of others' procrastination. Perhaps your boss knew a week ago that he wanted this project, but he just never got around to asking for it because he's been too "busy" to take the mere ten minutes it required to explain the project to you. So he dumps it over your head and wants it finished in one day. But in reality, it's going to take you a full three days to complete it. It's like the saying I've seen posted in photocopy shops: "Lack of planning on your part does not constitute an emergency on mine!"

▲ ▲ ▲

▼ ▼ ▼

▼ ENERGY BANDIT #5 | **Spending an inordinate amount of time perfecting menial tasks**

We can also get sucked into spending too much time on low-priority items. This is especially true of perfectionists, who can dig themselves deep into a given project to make sure every last little detail is just so. I heard a story about a couple who was removing wallpaper from their bathroom. The husband, a perfectionist, noted that they would have to remove the baseboards to remove all the wallpaper. The wife informed him that neither they, nor likely any future owners of the home, would want to remove the baseboards for any sane reason. And she promptly retrieved an X-Acto knife.

▲ ENERGY BOOSTER | **Keep the main thing the main thing**

Often we get sucked into performing tasks that don't add value. This is especially true in the workplace. We might have to write quarterly reports to our supervisors about the quarterly reports we submitted to another department. I know of a woman who worked as a fund-raiser for an organization. Her supervisor wanted her to spend several hours revising the output format of the report they reviewed in their weekly fund-raising meetings; he wanted it to be generated from the database instead of from a word-processing program. She politely asked whether he wanted her to spend four hours tweaking the report output format, which they spent less than an hour reviewing every week, or four hours calling donors to raise more money. He immediately saw her point.

Prioritizing is all about trimming the fat and avoiding expending too much effort on getting the little things just right. To minimize the time spent on every item you undertake, while still maintaining quality, try these methods of streamlining your energy into effortless efficiency.

- Do first what's due first.
- Try to resolve small items (requiring less than three minutes) immediately, without even writing them on your list. Just don't let all those tiny little items that pop up every day eat your entire schedule. Tend to the important or time-sensitive ones, and ditch the rest or tend to them later.
- Don't spend too much time on low-priority items. This will create a gridlock of high-priority items, all honking for your attention.
- Don't let perfectionism suck you too deeply into a minor task. Hence the saying "The perfect is the enemy of the good." Keep it in perspective. Be efficient. Set a limited time to accomplish the task. If you set aside only an hour to get it done, you'll get it done in an hour.

▲ ▲ ▲
▼ ▼ ▼

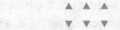

▼ ENERGY BANDIT #6 | **An inability to muster the energy needed to do chores**

Perhaps you're faced with tasks you dislike—they're redundant, they offer no challenge, and there's no inherent reward in accomplishing them, but you know you really should do them at some point. Annual household maintenance chores often fall into this category. So can filing in the office. Or filling out monthly activity reports.

▲ ENERGY BOOSTER | **Transform your outlook about truly necessary, but dreaded, tasks**

If you can't change the situation, then *change your mind*:

- Be grateful when things are easy. The task you have to accomplish may be redundant and offers zero intellectual stimulation—but if it's truly necessary, you can't blow it off. But it's much less stressful than having to deal with something that's difficult, such as a flat tire in the rain while on your way to a meeting with a prospective big client. Be glad when things are easy. Life is chock-full of difficult things. Enjoy whatever autopilot items come your way.

- Take the opportunity to make the task relaxing and meditative. Our lives are insanely busy. Think of a mindless task as a well-deserved respite from the hustle and bustle. Your boss wants you to stuff two hundred envelopes? No problem. It'll be a nice break from the annual budget that's been tying your brain into pretzels for the past five hours, not to mention giving your eyes a break from frying on the computer screen.

- Use your time and brainpower wisely. Focus your mind on something else while your body is on autopilot. When you're stuffing those envelopes, you just might be surprised that you've figured out the problem to that annual budget that's been plaguing you for days. Finish composing that poem in your head while you clean the sink. Brainstorm more effective and creative communication techniques for dealing with the kids. You'll be finished with your task before you realize it. I saw a sign once at a small airport that read, BOREDOM IS A CHOICE. It's so true. While performing a simple task, you can tie up any loose ends in your mind about other pressing details or think positive thoughts about yourself or a loved one.

▲ ▲ ▲

▼ ▼ ▼

▼ ENERGY BANDIT #7 | Procrastination

Call it putting things off, inactivity, or lack of initiative—no matter how you slice it, it is procrastination. The good news is that the dread of doing something is *always* worse than actually doing it. Procrastination builds stress, like a dam. But doing the thing transforms your energy, like a waterfall flowing.

▲ ENERGY BOOSTER | Force yourself to do it

When you finally do the task you've been putting off, the reward is the freedom from the stress that it was causing you. It feels so great to have it done. Good stuff immediately begins to flow into the space it was occupying. You're no longer paralyzed, and you get your energy back. If you keep procrastinating about doing something, it's still there, staring you in the face. But if you actually do it, it's gone; it's behind your back. If you're having trouble getting motivated, dangle a carrot in front of yourself. Tell yourself that as soon as you finish your fair share of the household chores, you can treat yourself to a square of dark chocolate. The flavonols are good for your heart, and it will curb your desire to do a face-dive into an entire cake. But don't exceed more than two or three squares per day!

▲ ▲ ▲
▼ ▼ ▼

▼ ENERGY BANDIT #8 | Doing the fun, easy, or trivial thing first

After I finish a speech, I get to the airport right away, even if my flight doesn't leave for some time. Clients have asked, "Would you like to camp out in this empty office after your presentation and do e-mail? You'll have plenty of time to get to the airport." I always politely decline, explaining that I can't truly relax until I'm at the airport and settled. Missing my plane is not worth the risk, so I put energy into getting to my gate (a rather difficult task with air travel these days), and then I can relax.

▲ ENERGY BOOSTER | **Work before play**

When you do the work first, it will no longer be hanging over your head. What fun is relaxation time if you've got a to-do list nagging at the back of your mind? After you accomplish your task, you can read your book, take a long, hot bath, watch the sunset, or whatever it is you love to do. Not only will this help you get it done, but it will help you get it done *faster* because you have something to look forward to. The earlier, the better. When faced with an unpleasant task such as arguing with your bank, dealing with an angry customer, or taking down outside Christmas lights, do it first thing in the morning. Otherwise, you'll lose energy thinking about it all day and probably will find an excuse not to do it.

▲ ▲ ▲

Thirteen

Time Management

Queen Elizabeth I of England, the most powerful, richest woman on earth at the time, is said to have whispered on her deathbed, "All my possessions for one moment of time." Time is your most valuable possession. To which tasks do you devote your most vigorous activity—and therefore your energy—every day? Do you waste your energy running in circles, feeling busy but not getting anywhere? You can be working hard to climb the big ladder of success, but you'll waste a lot of energy (and time) if you discover it's leaning on the wrong wall. An intense, personal commitment to achieve your goals gives you the vigor you need to move forward every day.

When you work on a task, your capacity to work on other tasks will slowly decline. When your energy is depleted, you don't work well until you catch your "second wind" and your energy is replenished once again. So you must select tasks purposefully, making sure the most important things get the lion's share of your energy and attention, before you run out of hours in the day. In this chapter, you'll look at the things that demand your attention and determine if you should be devoting so much of your energy to their completion. You'll ascertain your high-value activities, learn to set priorities, and find ways to eliminate demands that are merely in the way. Read on for ideas on how not to let the demands of time drain all your energy.

▼ ▼ ▼

▼ ENERGY BANDIT #1 | Having too much on your plate

If you've ever thought about how relaxing it would be if you were in jail right now, you're suffering from overwork. What is the definition of fatigue? A tombstone that says, "She finished everything on her to-do list." When you work nonstop, you don't have time to recharge your batteries and get ready for the next task. The Japanese use the word *karo jisatsu* to describe "death by overwork." Having too much on your plate and too many tasks than you can possibly accomplish can leave you feeling helpless. The reasons for overwork vary among personal, managerial, and organizational causes. Personally, you may have too much to do simply because you're not delegating enough (assuming you have someone to whom to delegate). Perhaps you feel so overwhelmed that you lack the time even to show someone how to help you. Expending energy on things that someone else is perfectly able to handle will leave you with less energy to focus on tasks of higher importance. Perhaps your boss isn't aware of how many things you need to do. You keep saying you have too much to do and not enough time to do it, but your complaints are falling on deaf ears. Organizationally, perhaps the reporting structure has you reporting to multiple "bosses" of sorts, requiring you to respond to people who aren't conducting your performance review. When conflicting priorities are thrown at you from all sides at once, it's very difficult to determine where to invest your energy.

▲ ENERGY BOOSTER | Practice purposeful abandonment

Eliminate anything on your to-do list that doesn't meet your goals and objectives or have long-term consequences for your work. The philosopher William James once wrote, "The art of being wise is the art of knowing what to overlook." Those high up in the corporate ranks usually have someone to be wise for them, by screening calls and e-mails, but everyone else is on their own. I worked with an administrative assistant who generated training reports every month for the operations group. She wasn't sure how the customer was using the reports, but they took her about four hours to create each month. I challenged her to call and ask. So she called and said, "We generate these reports for you, and we're happy to continue to do that, but we just wanted to check out its importance with you. Do you use it? Is it valuable?" It turned out the user did not review it monthly and really only needed a particular section of data from the report. After more discussion, they decided she would provide the report quarterly in a different summary format, saving hours of time and energy each month. Because she could eliminate the energy expenditure on that task, she had more time to focus on more worthwhile endeavors. It's important to keep the communication open with your "customer" and find out what really has value. Put a note in the e-mail text of the next report you send out and say, "Call me if you want to continue receiving this report." How many calls would you get? Would anyone notice if you stopped doing it? It's very humbling to do this and can be a big blow to your ego if you realize no one finds value in what you're providing. Celebrate. Now you can focus your energy on tasks that will result in greater recognition, and you can abandon things that don't add value.

▲ ▲ ▲
▼ ▼ ▼

▼ ENERGY BANDIT #2 | Trying to do everything yourself

When I first started my professional speaking business in 1992, I did everything myself. But I knew that if the business were to grow, I was going to have to stop going to the post office, making copies, and getting the copy machine repaired. So I hired my first employee in

1998, and after six years of flying solo, it was admittedly hard to let go.

▲ ENERGY BOOSTER | Get some help

As you change positions in your company, your level of delegation must shift if you are to have any time to yourself. You must become a leader instead of a doer and get work accomplished through other people. The great philosopher Virgil said long ago, "We are all not capable of everything." Never do anything that can be done just as well by someone who is paid less. If there is another person who can handle something you're doing, stop doing it. If someone can do the job 80 percent as well as you can, let that person do it. We mistakenly believe only we can do it correctly. Be open to new, innovative ways of tackling projects, and you will be pleased with the results. And you can focus your time on higher-value activities.

You should consider delegating the following types of work:

- Decisions you make most frequently and repetitively
- Assignments that will add variety to routine work
- Functions you dislike
- Work that will provide experience for employees
- Tasks that someone else is capable of doing
- Activities that will make a person more well rounded
- Tasks that will increase the number of people who can perform critical assignments
- Opportunities to use and reinforce creative talents
- Recurring matters
- Minor decisions
- Time-consuming details

You should always retain broader management duties such as overall planning, policy making, goal setting, and budget supervision, as well as tasks that involve confidential information or supervisor-subordinate relations. Make sure to monitor work, so you don't expend a lot of energy redoing things. I had an employee who was supposedly working a forty-hour week; when I checked the phone company logs, it turned out he was working for another company on the side and working for me only twenty hours a week. Don't be blind and assume even your "star" employee is giving you his or her best. I had another employee who was saying negative things about our company on myspace.com. Be tech-savvy and learn how to monitor Web sites that are visited.

▲ ▲ ▲
▼ ▼ ▼

▼ ENERGY BANDIT #3 | **Wasting time on nonproductive activities**

Do you ever get to the end of a day and wonder where the heck the time went? Fact is—you were robbed of precious minutes, and you're the biggest bandit of all. What activities weren't part of your agenda? Are you checking your eBay listings incessantly? Are you surfing the Internet, shopping for personal effects, when you should be writing a report? Are you leisurely reading blog postings when you have a project due tomorrow? Are you watching several hours of television a day? These are just a few examples of the way we focus our energy on things that waste time and then wonder why we didn't get anything done that we needed to accomplish that day. "But I was busy all day long," you lament. Yes, you were active, but you had no accomplishment, because you put effort toward things that ultimately had no value. Maybe you waste time through constructive procrastination: you clean out the kitchen cupboards when you should be paying bills and pay bills when you should be filling out tax forms. Yes, cleaning the cupboards is useful, but now you have to file an extension on your taxes.

▲ ENERGY BOOSTER | Focus on value

If you made a list of the top ten things you believe you're responsible for completing, asked your boss to do the same, and compared the two lists, would they be the same? If the answer is no, you are wasting your energy on things that ultimately don't matter in the eyes of your best customer. If your boss is the one who gives you performance reviews, it really doesn't matter what you think is important (although you usually have a better sense of this) if your boss doesn't value the results. It's a much wiser strategy to communicate with your boss about his or her expectations and discover what activities will yield the most significant praise—those are the things on which to spend your energy. If you truly feel you are understaffed and your boss is placing too many demands on your time that exceed your energy to complete them, try a time log. You can't simply complain: you must prove it. If you can show that every minute of every day is focused on high-value work, and you're still not getting it all done, then you have a case. Time logs are helpful, because we often don't write everything on our to-do list that we accomplish during the day. Once you see everything you did in black and white, you'll be shocked at how much you've accomplished. (*Bonus:* Send an e-mail to Timelog@TheProductivityPro.com and receive a time-log form and instructions for completion.)

▼ ENERGY BANDIT #4 | Biting off more than you can chew

I recently visited my grandparents and discovered a treasure trove of old family photographs. Especially precious were the ones of my mother as a little girl (none of which she had seen before) and my great-grandmother, whom I vaguely recall visiting before she passed away. With seven children, my grandparents had no idea how they were going to split the photos up after they passed, since many were one of a kind. My easy answer was to scan them, save them as .jpg files, and make CDs for each of my six uncles and my mother. So I packed my precious cargo in my suitcase and headed home. Then it hit me . . . what exactly did I get myself into? I counted the photos: 282. I quickly realized the huge time commitment and that although I was of course *able* to handle this task, I *shouldn't* handle it.

▲ ENERGY BOOSTER | **Outsource to a third party**

I pulled up my favorite freelance-for-hire site: www.elance.com. I posted my project requirements and received eighteen bids on my project, ranging anywhere from twenty-five cents to one dollar per scan. I awarded the project to a woman who took the time to e-mail me directly, tell me about her scanner, offer to complete a couple of test scans at different resolutions to test what printed best, and so forth. She quoted me seventy-five cents per scan, which was higher than some of the bids, but she suggested an enhancement to my project specs: upload the scans to a photo site as well, so that my relatives could order their own prints directly, and I wouldn't have to send them CDs myself. Even better.

How much do you spend going out to eat with your family? We can easily drop $75 on our family of five, especially if we order appetizers, dessert, and drinks. How much do you spend buying clothes or on entertainment? Put that money into hiring a housekeeper. At $240 a month, it's the best investment in my energy that I make. I have more time to spend with my kids, and I'd rather devote energy to them than to toilets. You just have to decide where your priorities are. Would you rather clean after work, or spend time with your family? Time with your loved ones is just like the Master-Card commercial: priceless.

Also think about how much your time is worth when you shop or choose a service provider. Let's say you want to purchase the latest $20 Harry Potter book. So you drive down to the local Barnes & Noble, park, find the book, wait in line, buy it, and drive home. That purchase could have taken an hour. So if you figure in the value of your time at $20 an hour, the book would cost double the price. Buy it on barnesandnoble.com, spend five minutes, pay $4.50 for shipping, and the total cost is less than $30. You just saved money. Always add in the dollar value of your time to transactions. If you make $50 an hour, a $.75 coupon is not worth your time to clip unless you can cut it out, save it, find it on shopping day, and hand it to the clerk in fifty-four seconds.

▲ ▲ ▲
▼ ▼ ▼

▼ ENERGY BANDIT #5 | Multitasking and lack of focus

A study in multitasking by Morton Christiansen, associate professor of psychology at Cornell University, who coauthored the study with Christopher Conway, a National Institutes of Health research fellow at Indiana University (*Psychological Science*, October 2006), reported that people can multitask fairly well when they use different senses to complete tasks. For example, you can drive while keeping an eye on traffic and listening to the radio at the same time, or chop up vegetables while you're talking on the phone. However, similar stimuli competing for the same senses at the same time—such as two people talking to you at once—jam your perceptual frequencies. That's why, as parents, we've always intuitively said, "One at a time, please." Humans learn "sequential structure from multiple sources at the same time, as long as the sensory characteristics of the sources do not overlap," Christiansen said. So if you're trying to pay attention to two different technologies at once, your brain slows to a crawl, and it takes an inordinate amount of energy to attempt to concentrate.

▲ ENERGY BOOSTER | **Do one thing at a time**

The challenge is that our work tasks all tend to be on the same frequency: they require our conscious thought. You have twenty-seven things on your to-do list, and you're either tackling them in the order you think of them or by what you feel like doing, not necessarily by priority. You start in on a task and suddenly remember to tell a coworker about a change in a project. So you get up, walk down the hall to talk with him, stop off in the break room for a cup of tea, run into your friend, and chat for a while. Then you decide you might as well use the bathroom and read the postings on the bulletin board when you come out. When you arrive at your coworker's office, he's not there, so you make your way back to your office, open your e-mail to send him a note—oooh, seventeen new messages. You spend an hour on e-mail and then think, "What was I working on?" If this is a typical pattern in your day, you must stop jumping back and forth between activities without any focus. You just consumed a lot of time, used up a lot of your available energy on low-priority tasks, and still did not complete your original, important task.

Many people mistakenly think that doing several things at once improves their productivity. Not so, say Rubinstein and Meyer, authors of "Human Perception and Performance" (*Journal of Experimental Psychology*, August 2001), who proved that multitasking, in fact, *reduces* productivity. Their research determined that for all types of tasks, subjects lost time when they had to switch from one task to another. Multitasking involves deciding to switch tasks, making the switch, and then getting warmed up on what you switched to or switched back to. For example, let's say you're banging away on a report on your computer. Then the phone rings and you answer it. When you hang up, there is a lag between returning to your document, where you say, "Okay, where was I?" and getting your train of thought back. In effect, you briefly get "writer's block" as you go from one task to the other.

Try these tips to help you stay put and work through a task:

- Protect your time. When you need to focus on a task, try to prevent interruptions if possible, such as by closing your door or working in a conference room.
- Start with clear, achievable goals. For example, "Here are the two most important things I need to accomplish today."
- Break tasks down into manageable pieces. For example, "First I will work on the report. Then I will make my airline reservations."
- Write down thoughts but don't obey them. When your memory serves you up a reminder, don't follow the rabbit trail. Just capture the note on your to-do list and go right back to what you were doing. For example, "Did I remember to fax that supply order? Wait, nope, do not handle that right now . . . let me just write it down here so I remember to check later."
- Get organized. "I need the meeting notes from last week. The spreadsheet from Karen." Have everything around you and ready to go, so you don't go looking for it in e-mail and get sidetracked.
- Focus and get to it. Don't let low-priority activities—such as making personal plans or chatting—stand in the way of accomplishing critical tasks. Say something like, "Can I call you at four o'clock to talk about the concert tickets?"

▲ ▲ ▲

▼ ▼ ▼

| **Lack of desire**

Despite decades of research and theorizing, the subject of human motivation remains contested. Motivation is all about energy. You sometimes lack the energy or desire to work on something you know you should. Perhaps you've put in too many hours previously with very little reward, and because of your disappointment or disillusion, you're unmotivated to keep up the pace. Maybe you dislike a particular task, either because you can do it in your sleep or because it's so daunting you don't know where to start. Perhaps you're not given enough authority to accomplish your work, your work isn't acknowledged in ways you feel good about, or you have little input into decisions that affect your work. Whatever the cause, lack of motivation toward your work is a psychological energy drain that needs immediate attention.

▲ ENERGY BOOSTER | **Be disciplined**

When you promise someone you will complete a task by a certain time, do you do it? Or does the deadline slip past once again, with you muttering to yourself, "Stupid. What is wrong with you?" Now you aren't able to focus on anything, always aware of this dark cloud hanging over your head. Guilt sucks the energy right out of you. Instead, decide today that you are going to be a person of your word—someone others can count on. Seek to control yourself. If you say to yourself, "I probably shouldn't be doing this right now," you're probably right. If you're honest with yourself, how many hours could you save every day by being more disciplined? And could you leave the office earlier with that saved time? If tomorrow you arrived at work and *didn't* get a cup of coffee . . . *didn't* go on the Internet . . . *didn't* talk to your friend . . . *didn't* get your new blog postings . . . *didn't* get sucked into e-mail for ninety minutes . . . *what* could you use that energy on instead that will make you proud of yourself and give you a boost of satisfaction for the entire day? When you finally complete the task, the freedom from the stress it was causing you is its own reward. Good things begin to flow into the space the negative guilt used to occupy. You're no longer paralyzed, and you get your energy back.

▲ ▲ ▲
▼ ▼ ▼

▼ ENERGY BANDIT #7 | Maintaining the status quo

Yes, it's important to maintain your systems: food is prepared, the house is cleaned, dishes are washed, bills are paid, and so forth. But nothing is gained with those activities; there is no forward momentum. Those things are done simply to keep you from sliding backward. You got out all the nice china for Thanksgiving dinner. You washed it. You ate on it. You washed it. You put it away. Back to the same place you were before. Yes, of course you have wonderful memories with your family and relaxed a bit. But your situation is the same.

▲ ENERGY BOOSTER | Make some progress

Understand the difference between maintenance and progress. Tidying up the living room is maintenance. Cleaning and conditioning the leather furniture is progress. So, each day, ask, "Did I make any progress?" Did you take the time to organize an area? Get a family photo taken? Go through your kids' playroom and give away a bunch of stuff they never play with? Map out the shelving project in your garage? NOW your condition is improved, and your situation is different. You have made progress. When your guests have left and everything's back in order (maintained), you're back to "normal."

Then work on some progress tasks: wrap gifts, get holiday shopping done, or organize a drawer. Some people skip the maintenance and go directly to progress tasks, which can be okay too, unless you're like me and feel a bit unsettled when surrounded by clutter or incompletions. So get everything back in order as quickly as possible, so you have time for new projects. To experience forward momentum, don't think "Done," think "Get back to normal" and then "NEXT."

▲ ▲ ▲
▼ ▼ ▼

▼ ENERGY BANDIT #8 | Trying to get it all done

When is the last time you put your head on the pillow at the end of the day and exclaimed, "I'm DONE!"? Probably never. And you probably never will.

▲ ENERGY BOOSTER | Realize that your to-do list is never going to end—until you're dead

There will always be more things to do than time to do them. There will always be a constant, never-ending stream of things coming at you: it's called life. That's okay—what would you do with yourself if your to-do list *did* end? Even the wealthiest people have to feed themselves and dress themselves. You're alive; therefore, you have things to do. Think about it: superwealthy people either destroy themselves with chronic complaining about mere trifles or get the most mileage from their freedom by making the world a better place through volunteering and giving. Sophia Loren, who has enough money to pay a large staff of people to wait on her hand and foot, once remarked that you should do something practical every day. No, this doesn't mean that you should feel obliged to busybody around 24–7. But it does mean that there's no way of completely escaping a few practical tasks every day, no matter how minute they are. Descartes said, "I think, therefore I am." We can add to that, "I am, therefore I do."

Don't work half-crazed each day, fooling yourself that you can actually get everything done. It's like shoveling the driveway before it stops snowing—it's fruitless. Think of it this way: will your children remember when they're grown and gone that you didn't mop the kitchen floor for two weeks in 2004, or will they remember the time you took them skiing on a Saturday afternoon? If something on your to-do list is bothering you, ask yourself, "Will this be important next week?"

▲ ▲ ▲

Fourteen

Learning

Your energy level isn't entirely dependent on your physical condition, or even your emotional and psychological health. One of the biggest energy stealers is a lack of mental and intellectual stimulation. There's a good reason an exciting book can tempt you to read well past your bedtime, while a boring book will put you to sleep (which is why I'm hoping you're not sawing logs right about now). The same dull environment, experienced the same way every day for months on end, can bore you to tears.

Take a look at yourself. Is *your* life the same every single day? Do you feel like a robot, just going through the motions? If you feel like you're wasting your energy because you're unchallenged and uninspired, then you're probably right. There's a good reason the saying "Grow or die" is something of a cliché, because it verbalizes a deep-rooted truth about human nature: that *you need to keep growing intellectually all the days of your life.*

I'm not just talking about education here, at least in terms of getting a degree so that you'll be more employable (although that's great too); there's much more to it than that. If you want your brain to continue to serve you well into old age, you have to keep it active. A long-term study of a population of nuns in Mankato, Minnesota, has revealed that the ones who keep themselves mentally active not only live longer but also suffer the lowest levels of dementia, Alzheimer's disease, and other ailments of the brain and memory that commonly strike in old age.[1]

In this chapter, you'll be encouraged to challenge yourself every day and learn continuously. I'll throw out a bunch of ideas about learning new things, growing intellectually, doing puzzles, reading new genres, taking classes, and getting back into life again. Mental stimulation is exercise for the brain, and if it's lacking, you'll end up with the mental equivalent of flab.

▼ ▼ ▼

▼ ENERGY BANDIT #1 | A lack of challenges

Think back to the days when you first learned to drive. You were nervous but alert while under instruction, and your first few solo drives were probably fraught with moments of sheer terror. You certainly weren't bored. For months, you focused pretty tightly on the matter at hand, and even if you had a passenger, you probably paid more attention to the road than to that person.

Flash forward to today. You pretty much get into your car, fasten your seatbelt, start the engine, and away you go. Everything is so familiar and rote that it all becomes automatic. Concentration is no longer a concern, and unless some idiot does something stupid in front of you, it becomes boring. Ever heard of highway hypnosis? That's when the task of driving becomes so simple, and the environment so predictable, that you're bored out of your skull. You're watching the road, and your body is doing everything it's supposed to when it's supposed to do it, but your mind is elsewhere—and suddenly you've gone fifty miles and don't remember how you got there.

A recent survey by Korn/Ferry International, a leading executive recruitment firm, cited "lack of challenges" as a prime reason why business executives changed jobs. In fact, it topped the list at 33 percent, well ahead of the 20 percent who cited "ineffective leadership" as their exit reason.[2]

▲ ENERGY BOOSTER | Challenge yourself to learn something new every day

How can you be anything but bored if you don't learn something new occasionally? Human knowledge is so vast and complex that there's *always* something new to be learned. Most physicians and scientists become specialists in order to really understand a specific corner of their field, and to potentially make contributions there.

Learning is great for your brain. A report in the journal *American Scientist* explained that when the brain discovers something—and says "aha"—it receives a dose of what equates to natural opium. When you learn something new, your brain is washed by a cascade of biochemicals.[3] Make sure you learn something new every day. For example, you could learn a new word every day. Will you ever really need to know what *onomatopoeia* means? Maybe not, but you never know. Just learning the word stretches a mental muscle or two.

You don't have to take on something too difficult—like a foreign language or a new programming code—too quickly, or you may feel anxious due to your lack of ability and shut down. You want to learn in the range of what Mihaly Csikszentmihalyi of the University of Chicago described as "flow," where your ability to perform and concentrate is greatly enhanced.[4] Csikszentmihalyi describes the "competency zone," where your abilities and the task are in alignment. Below that zone, you're bored. Too far outside that zone, you become less effective due to your inability to perform and the subsequent energy drain. The trick with learning something new is to push yourself a *little* bit outside the zone, so you learn, but not far enough that you despair and give up.

▲   ▲   ▲

▼ ▼ ▼

▼ ENERGY BANDIT #2 | Few creative outlets in your life

There's a reason that the zeal to create is often referred to as "creative *energy*." Channeling some of your time into creating something—whether it's a meal, a watercolor, or a poem—can help you unwind.

▲ ENERGY BOOSTER | Exercise your creativity

You don't have to be a James Beard to enjoy cooking, or a Renoir to enjoy painting. You could write novels or look for rare bugs or learn to blow glass in your spare time. You might find that you're a whiz at building ships in a bottle or drawing cartoons, or singing Guns N' Roses songs. Even if you're not, you can have a lot of fun trying.

In 2006, my hometown of Denver, Colorado, experienced a giant blizzard two days before Christmas and another the week after Christmas. The storms closed the airport repeatedly and spoiled the holiday plans of thousands. With all the snow, the city was forced to slow (and shut) down. The people who weren't stuck in the airport unexpectedly spent several days holed up with their families. My sons love to build Bionicle, Lego, and Exo-Force kits. I'd never tried assembling these kits before—all the little pieces and detailed instructions seemed so complicated—but I had lots of time to figure it out. So I gave it a shot . . . and discovered I really enjoyed it. It was real quality time with my sons doing an activity they love. Now we display the completed figures in their bedroom bookcases and enjoy looking at them and talking about the experience we had building them together.

▲ ▲ ▲

▼ ▼ ▼

▼ ENERGY BANDIT #3 | Feeling like your life is a treadmill: not going anywhere

If your day-to-day routine seems mind-numbingly dull, it's because, well, *it is*. You've had so much practice at what you're doing that you're really good at it; suddenly, everything is too easy. As with the driving example earlier, if there's no surprise left, and little more that you can accomplish, you're going to lose interest—and you'll find it difficult to devote any energy at all to those little tasks that keep you on track.

▲ ENERGY BOOSTER | Make a drastic change in your life

Sometimes it takes a major shift in the landscape of your life to revive your interest in the world to the point where it's worth the trouble to get out of bed. If, after a long look at your career, you find that your work doesn't make good use of your abilities, consider changing jobs. We've all experienced the extreme focus and sense of concentration that comes with starting a new job: you're energetic and more aware of everything around you, because you're concerned with making a good impression and doing well in your new environment. This goes back to the whole concept of learning new things. You don't need to change your career completely, but the combination of a new setting and new, unfamiliar challenges will probably have you buzzing along with a level of energy that you probably thought was lost to you.

You could also go back to school full-time and get a degree. Most professors enjoy dealing with older students, because they realize (1) that they're serious about learning; and (2) that they're mature enough not to complain about their assignments all the time. It's hard to fall into a lackluster rut when you're attending full-time college classes because the scenery changes with every new semester. Not only are you undertaking new and different tasks with every individual class, but you'll find yourself moving on to something more advanced every few months (ideally, anyway). Constant learning can't help but stretch your mental abilities on a continual basis, and what you've learned can always be applied later in your career. It's never too late to go back to school, especially in these days of longer life spans; in fact, older adults are doing it more than ever before. Despite the cost and other drawbacks, it's a great way to keep your mind healthy.

Another big change to try is moving, which is an extreme way to break out of a rut, but it will definitely expand your mental-energy horizons. Like changing jobs, picking up and moving your residence can shake you up enough to restart your interest in life and, in so doing, revivify you energetically. You needn't go far. Even if you don't change towns or jobs, dealing with all the details of finding a new place, getting everything packed, moving, unpacking, and learning the ins and outs of your new neighborhood can't help but perk you up, at least for a while. Such a radical change may prove stressful, of course, but you have to consider the options: would you rather be sunk in boredom or depression, or would you rather be alert, energetic, and slightly stressed? It's your call.

▼ ENERGY BANDIT #4 | **Never cracking open a book**

Even if you're not learning a single new thing, reading offers a variety of benefits that can help you discharge any negative energy and recharge with the good kind. Among other things, reading gives you the following:

- An escape from your daily routine
- General relaxation
- Stress relief
- Stimulation for the right side of your brain (the analytical side)
- Entertainment
- Enjoyment
- Mental and physical rejuvenation[5]

▲ ENERGY BOOSTER | **Challenge yourself to read more**

Reading will take you to places you've never been, letting you vicariously (and safely) experience things you may never get to do in real life. In our culture, reading is a necessary life skill, and that's more than most forms of entertainment can offer. It may be a passive exercise as far as physical activity goes, but it is a vigorous mental exercise. The most predictable potboiler can keep your emotions engaged and your mind active, and can serve as a distraction from your workaday worries. It can also expand your horizons and contribute significantly to your education.

If you're already a devoted reader and you're still down in the dumps, try adding different genres to your repertoire. If you're a sci-fi junkie, for example, read a mystery or two, or even a western. Even if you happen to pick a novel that most readers in the genre would find old hat, it will probably be new to you. If you're bored with fiction in general, try nonfiction. A nonfiction blockbuster like Mark Kurlansky's *Cod* (which really is about cod) can be as fascinating as a well-researched mystery; Sebastian Junger's *The Perfect Storm* grips just as tightly as a Ludlum thriller; Donald and Petie Kladstrup's *Wine and War: The French, the Nazis, and the Battle for France's Greatest Treasure* describes the French's daring, dangerous acts of Nazi resistance, and is sure to send your heart racing.

▼ ▼ ▼

▼ ENERGY BANDIT #5 | Lack of mental stimulation and training

Fortunately, in our modern world, you won't have much of a problem finding something to stimulate your intellectual capacity. If you can't keep yourself mentally active in the ordinary course of your tasks, then find something to stretch the boundaries of your mind whenever you can. It may do more than save your job—it may help you live longer. Remember the nuns of Mankato? Not only do they have fewer brain problems as they age, but they have greater longevity than most people; reaching the age of ninety is not unusual for them, and some make it into their hundreds. According to those who study them, it's because they spurn an idle mind as the devil's plaything, and spend their time quizzing each other, debating various issues, doing puzzles, and writing in journals. Those who earn college degrees and teach also tend to live longer. More than one hundred of the Mankato nuns have donated their brains to science upon their deaths, and the researchers who have examined them claim that the brains of the more active nuns display more interconnections between neural cells, so that they had bigger "backup systems" available in the event that some of their neural pathways failed.

▲ ENERGY BOOSTER | Do puzzles to sharpen your mind

Just as reading can kick-start your intellectual energy level, so can puzzles. I'm not just talking about jigsaw puzzles here, although those can aid with concentration, topographical skills, and associational abilities. Verbal and written puzzles also come highly recommended. They're often known as brainteasers, and for good reason—they stretch the imagination, make us rethink assumptions, and often help us connect disparate facts we might not otherwise have considered related.

Try your hand at different types of puzzles, until you find one that suits you:

- The flowering of literacy over the past few centuries has made possible a new type of puzzle: the word puzzle, exemplified by the crossword and the acrostic. These puzzles require a fairly extensive level of cultural and literary knowledge, and in the right hands can be extremely complex and difficult (*New York Times* crosswords are notoriously hard). You can try them on your computer at www.bestcrosswords.com.

- Sudoku (my absolute favorite) is a numerical puzzle that has gained popularity in America. I keep a book of Sudoku puzzles in my briefcase. When I'm flying, I have a ritual of working on a puzzle until we take off, at which time I switch to real work on my computer. Sudoku was invented in America years ago but first hit it big in Japan before sloshing back across the pond to ring cash registers here. Like chess, the rules are simple; you can learn them in a few minutes, but it'll take awhile to master this kind of puzzle—they can be wickedly hard. If you'd like to sharpen your mind against the whetstone of Sudoku, you can start at www.websudoku.com. Good luck!

- If you get good at Sudoku, you can try your luck against the harder Kakuro, which is like Sudoku on steroids. This is my father's favorite addiction; he will sit in a chair for hours completing a puzzle. He says he gets so engaged and absorbed that time seems to fly.

▲ ▲ ▲

▼ ▼ ▼

▼ ENERGY BANDIT #6 | Not pushing yourself to grow and learn

You've been there, done that. Gone around the block a few times. Been in your job for many years and can do it with your eyes closed. Sometimes we get a little apathetic and jaded, thinking that we don't have much to learn. In most aspects of life, you can't afford apathy. This is especially the case in your job, because you want to be perceived as a team player who cares about your own fate and the fate of the company. This is less of a problem if you're the boss, but you do have to care enough to keep coming to work every day and doing the things you need to do to make your business a success.

▲ ENERGY BOOSTER | Get a mentor

For many of us, developing new personal relationships is a great way to go to the next level. Consider acquiring a mentor to help you with what you're going through. Several years ago, I approached Dianna Booher, CSP, CPAE, whom I'd been watching for many years at National Speakers Association conferences, and asked her to be my mentor—well, I guess I didn't *exactly* ask, I just kept requesting thirty minutes to speak with her once a month until it became a ritual. Working with Dianna has helped me grow my business and avoid the pitfalls that come with my particular career of speaking and authorship. She has guided me around some big potholes and time wasters on my road to success. Find someone who is where you want to be in ten years. I had read many of her books (she has written more than forty-five to date) and sat in her educational breakout sessions (www.booher.com). I admired her so much and wanted to emulate her in my career. There's more to achievement than just barreling up the ladder of advancement, and a good mentor will provide you with the tips and guidance you need. Your mentor may also know tricks to help you revive your interest in your career or life. Our relationship has turned into a wonderful friendship as well, and I think of her as my second mom in many ways. Be sure to show appreciation for your mentor every time you receive the gift of time from that person. Thank-you notes, expressions of gratitude, and small gifts are especially appropriate.

▲ ▲ ▲
▼ ▼ ▼

▼ ENERGY BANDIT #7 | Not contributing to the greater good

Work, home, sleep. Work, home, sleep. Does this cycle seem to repeat itself day in and day out? Most of us like having some structure to our lives, but too much quickly becomes dull. Having to deal with the same old same old every single day can really drag you down. If you're feeling lethargic and trapped in a cycle of inactivity, perhaps you need to do something bigger than yourself.

▲ ENERGY BOOSTER | Get involved in a worthy cause

Another way to break out of your everyday routine is to give your time to a worthy cause. Volunteering is a great way to help make the world a better place. Depending on what you're interested in volunteering for, it can also help you realize how good you've got it in life. These questions can help you decide how to contribute:

- What issues are you interested in? Reading to children at the library? Making audio recordings of the daily newspaper for the blind? Helping a local environmental group with water-quality monitoring? Feeding the hungry? Finding homes for abandoned animals? Being a volunteer firefighter?

- Look at your schedule to see how often you can volunteer. A couple of hours a week? A couple of hours a month? All day every Monday?

There are literally hundreds of such causes out there, so you can easily match at least one to your interests. If you like building things, consider Habitat for Humanity, where you'll be in good company—former president Jimmy Carter participates. If you like kids, consider becoming a Big Brother or Big Sister. If you like cooking, volunteer at a soup kitchen. The possibilities are endless, and despite the fact that you're volunteering, you'll still get paid—not in money but in good feeling, which will permeate and brighten all aspects of your life. What a great way to inject more energy into your day.

If you're raring to volunteer, but you're having trouble choosing a cause to volunteer for, here's a great matching service to try: http://www.volunteermatch.org/.

▲ ▲ ▲
▼ ▼ ▼

▼ ENERGY BANDIT #8 | **Staying inside your comfort zone**

Do you make time to develop friendships in your neighborhood? Or do you drive down the street, hit the garage-door opener, drive in, and close it behind you—never to actually interact with any of your neighbors?

▲ ENERGY BOOSTER | **Make new friends**

I remember the old Girl Scout saying "Make new friends, but keep the old, one is silver and the other gold." There's no need to snub your old friends, but a few new faces in your personal circle can add a bit of needed spice to your life. Extending yourself can be a little bit difficult for the introverted among us, but it's a relatively simple way to recharge your life. Humans are social animals; we need to relate with other people on a continual basis to avoid the boring void of anomie. This becomes especially important as you age; every new friend (however informal) means a new link in your personal network, a new tie to keep you anchored to reality and all its exciting potential.[6]

You don't have to hang out in bars to meet new friends (unless, of course, that's your style). You can also join a writer's group, a reading circle, a hobby club, a church, or what have you. Play bridge once a week with a group of friends. Join a quilting circle. Go for daily walks with a friend. Go out to eat with a group of friends once a week. Talk to your best friend on the phone once a day. You can keep in touch several times a week via e-mail too. But don't let e-mail replace telephone contact; you need to hear another live human voice to prevent loneliness from creeping in.

▲ ▲ ▲

Part Three
PERIPHERY

Fifteen

Environment

Periphery quiz item #15:
Will you people be quiet so I can think?

Does your environment boost or bust your energy? How do lighting, decor, smell, noise level, temperature, ergonomics, and color affect you? Spending hours in front of a computer can literally be a pain, and workplace injuries can be severe. If your back hurts from a bad chair, for example, you'll exert more energy to maintain the same concentration level as before, so you'll fatigue and run out of energy more quickly than usual. Even certain smells can reduce stress and anxiety. Lighting levels are directly linked to mood: as much as 10 percent of the population is affected by the short days of winter, which cause them to crave high-carbohydrate foods. Noise is another factor: Cornell University researchers found that children in schools bombarded by frequent aircraft noise don't learn to read as well as children in quiet schools. Low-level noise in open-style offices results in higher levels of stress and lower task motivation.

In this chapter, you'll learn about these issues and how to assess the impact of your environment. You'll discover how some simple changes can boost your energy. I'll show you some straightforward techniques—such as using music, scents, blue light, and headsets—to make your space more refreshing.

▼ ▼ ▼

▼ ENERGY BANDIT #1 | **Physical discomfort at your desk**

It's really hard to concentrate and be productive when you're hurt-ing. Working can be a real pain in the neck—and in the back, and the wrists, and the legs, and the eyes too. Bad posture, badly de-signed furniture, and poor work habits can generate enough discom-fort to damage your health. When you're in pain, you're forced to use more fuel on less work. While blue-collar and outdoor jobs of-fer a multitude of opportunities for physical discomfort and injury, the culprits in offices are usually furniture: poorly designed chairs, desks that are too high or too low, and especially keyboards, com-puter or otherwise.

▲ ENERGY BOOSTER | **Make sure that your workspace is ergonomically designed**

The term *ergonomic* refers to healthy workspace setups. As used in most work settings, it refers primarily to the physical environment, particularly furniture and work tools. It doesn't matter if you're a cabbie or an office worker; you need comfortable furniture and tools to keep your energy and productivity up, especially if you're doing repetitive tasks like typing all day. Yet you may simply become ac-customed to your discomfort, even as it siphons off your creative and physical energy. That's a mistake, because making your work-space more ergonomic will not only increase your own comfort, it can also be more profitable for both you and your company.[1] Try these adjustments:

- Wipe out lower back pain. Chairs with adjustable back support and properly sized desks result in less discomfort for the user, which translates into greater productivity and a better use of your available energy reserves. Choose a correct chair that allows you good back support and lets your legs relax at a 90-degree angle with your feet flat on the floor. Don't cross your legs at the knees, which can lead to varicose veins. Before purchasing a chair, check with the American National Standards Institute, which has developed standards for office chairs.

- If you're trying to type while talking on the phone, don't cradle the phone between your jaw and shoulder. This can lead to neck tension and TMJ jaw problems. If you have to spend a lot of time on the phone, use a headset instead. They're inexpensive and work great.

- Support your wrists with specially designed pads at the base of your keyboard and on your mouse to prevent carpal tunnel syndrome. A mouse station placed slightly lower than desk level will help prevent shoulder tension. And resist the temptation to leave your hand on the mouse constantly; remove it regularly and rotate it, especially if the computer takes more than a few seconds to complete its operation.

▲ ▲ ▲
▼ ▼ ▼

▼ ENERGY BANDIT #2 | Repetitive motion injuries

RMIs are caused by doing the same thing over and over again: typing, swinging a tennis racket, tapping away on your BlackBerry, and the like. Following are some common RMIs:

- *Tennis elbow (a.k.a. lateral epicondylitis):* an irritation of the tendons that flex the fingers, at their attachment at the inside of the elbow
- *Golfer's elbow (medial epicondylitis):* an irritation of the tendons that extend the fingers, at their attachment at the outside of the elbow

- **Trigger finger:** a jerkiness of the fingers caused by irritation of the tendons in the hand
- **Bursitis:** irritation of the bursae, usually over major joints such as the knee
- **Carpal tunnel syndrome:** pain, numbness, tingling, and weakness of the hands caused by the pinching of the hand's median nerve, generally because of hand placement and posture while keyboarding. Having to hold your wrists at unnatural angles all day while your hands dance over the keys can result in repetitive motion injuries that may not only be extremely painful but can, in certain situations, cut your productivity to nil.

Depending on its severity, an RMI can either sap your energy because of your need to focus beyond the discomfort or wreck your productivity altogether by sidelining you. The best way to deal with RMIs is through the "ounce of prevention" method by not getting them at all. It's truly amazing how easy it is to ignore our own physical symptoms of overuse or overwork and let the pain become "normal" or dull. Take it from me—use your pain as a signal that something's wrong and listen to your body.

▲ ENERGY BOOSTER | **Mix up your moves**

I once developed a mysterious pain in my right hand and went to the doctor. My smart doc asked me how much time I spent on the computer, and after hearing my answer, suggested it could be my mouse. I doubted it, because I had recently acquired a newfangled, ergonomically correct mouse. But wanting to be a good patient, I purchased an old-fashioned, small mouse. Within days—voilà!—my thumb stopped hurting. It turned out that the "ergonomically correct" mouse was too big for my hand. Because I actually had to grasp the left side of it, rather than just laying my hand over the top, it made my hand ache.

Next, my thumb began to hurt. Diagnosis? "BlackBerry thumb," which is a "repetitive stress injury characterized by swelling and pain at the base of the thumb and caused by prolonged use of the thumb while operating a BlackBerry or other personal digital assistant."[2] Well, now I'm not laughing so loud.

More recently, I went to a hand surgeon with a severe, stabbing pain at the base of my thumb and wrist. I left after a diagnosis of tendonitis, a cortisone shot in the joint, a wrist brace to sleep in for one month, and a strict admonishment to not hold my handheld phone and type e-mail with the same hand.

If you're having a nagging pain, see your doctor and determine what behaviors might be causing it.

▲ ▲ ▲
▼ ▼ ▼

▼ ENERGY BANDIT #3 | Bad lighting

Good ergonomic design means more than just good furniture; though that's an important start, you must also pay attention to the other items in your environment. Think of your five senses, and determine how much better you perform when each is functioning within its prime operating range. Unless you're the boss or you own your own business, it's unlikely that there's much you can do about the general design of your workplace. You can, however, endeavor to surround yourself with the right lighting.

▲ ENERGY BOOSTER | Create a well-lit office space

Good lighting is more important than most of us realize, though its value is clear if you think about it a little. One way that good lighting can help is obvious: if the ambient light level is sufficient, you can get your job done with less eyestrain. Like low-level physical pain, excessive eyestrain will force you to expend more energy to concentrate, leaving you wrung out at the end of the day. But there may be other ways in which lighting can affect a person's energy level: recent workplace research suggests that nothing beats natural lighting for spurring productivity. Natural sunlight contains blue light, which most artificial lighting lacks, and some researchers believe that it's that blue light that sparks greater energy in workers.[3] At a certain level this makes sense, as humans lived and worked in natural lighting for many thousands of years before artificial lighting was invented. However, the jury is still out on the issue of blue light's effectiveness, and the research is silent on why fluorescent lighting (which is noticeably bluish) doesn't have the same effect. Regardless, office fluorescent lights that constantly flicker can act as a stimulant that saps energy. It's best to switch to full-spectrum lighting or sit by a window whenever you can. One worker told me she disconnected one of the two fluorescent tubes above her workstation, which made it easier to see the computer monitor.

▼ ENERGY BANDIT #4 | A distracting office environment, with too many things clamoring for your attention

If you smell something disgusting, you have to use energy to pay attention to it and figure out what it is. If you're too hot or too cold, it's hard to concentrate on your work.

▲ ENERGY BOOSTER | **Strive for a neutral background**

The goal is to not have anything around that your body has to use energy either to pay attention to or to avoid paying attention to. Consider these environmental factors:

- **Smell.** You can use energy trying to ignore unpleasant odors, especially if a smell actually makes you sick to your stomach. And it's not just the unpleasant odors like stinky feet and old food in the company fridge that can affect you: we've all been exposed to our coworkers' ideas of acceptable scents, from the special Indonesian coffee that's passed through civet cat digestive tracts[4] to cologne worn in knock-you-down concentrations. It's enough to make some people sue,[5] but a better idea is to try to fight fire with fire. If you can replace or cover up the smell, do so; incense, a scented candle (if allowed in your workplace), or an air freshener might do the trick. Research indicates that some smells, like lavender, cut grass, and pine trees, can actually help to reduce stress, which is the reasoning behind aromatherapy. It might also be a good idea to purchase an inexpensive air cleaner to run in your workspace, if the offensive odor is one that will respond to it.

- **Temperature.** It's probably no surprise to you that temperature can make a difference in your energy level and productivity; after all, you use up a lot of energy shivering (since the whole point is to raise your body temperature), and it's hard to get a lot done when you're trembling all the time. But even at more reasonable temperature levels, you're likely to accomplish more when you're warmer. A recent study revealed that when the thermostat was raised from 68 degrees to 77 degrees, worker output increased by about 10 percent, to the tune of about two dollars per hour per employee.[6] It seems unlikely that this trend would continue much above

80°F, since once again physical discomfort would become a factor, this time from overheating.

- *Color.* Investigate the link between color and worker productivity, and you'll keep coming across the name of Dr. Nancy Kwallek, director of the interior design program at the University of Texas at Austin's School of Architecture. In a recent study, she had workers do mundane clerical tasks in offices with several different color schemes and discovered that white is absolutely the worst color for productivity—at first. After being exposed to an all-white environment for a while, most workers adjusted just fine. For those who could screen out their environment from the beginning, however, bright colors were more effective, since they seem to stimulate people in general. Those more easily distracted by the environment did better in rooms painted a cooler color, like blue-green. Ultimately, however, the most effective color scheme was a mix of the two: blue-green over soft red, separated by wood paneling (wainscoting).[7]

▲ ▲ ▲
▼ ▼ ▼

▼ ENERGY BANDIT #5 | Improper computer setup and usage

Regardless of your field of work, chances are you spend at least a few hours sitting in front of a computer every day. With a few common-sense measures, you can protect your overall energy and your long-term productivity.

▲ ENERGY BOOSTER | Limit your overexposure to electromagnetic radiation

While there's nothing wrong with a little electromagnetic radiation—after all, that's what sunlight and radio waves are—it's a bad idea to get too much of it. Most of our commonplace electronic devices emit varying levels of radiation, and our computer monitors are the worst culprits. Here are a few guidelines to keep in mind:

- Be sure your monitor conforms to MPRII guidelines established by the Swedish National Board of Testing. This ensures that the electromagnetic fields are at significantly lower levels than those emitted by older models.
- Stay an arm's length away from the screen. Stay four feet from the back and the sides of the screen, as that's where electromagnetic fields are strongest. Note that walls do not absorb these electromagnetic fields, so be aware of computer arrangements in adjacent rooms.
- Turn off your computer when you're not using it to reduce electromagnetic radiation.[8]
- Don't be a hypochondriac about your computer's electromagnetic radiation; your mental stress about it is much more harmful!

▼ ENERGY BANDIT #6 | Eyestrain

Itching, irritated, blurry eyes make it difficult to dedicate your energy to worthwhile pursuits. Staring continually at a computer screen that's too close to you can quickly give you a headache.

▲ ENERGY BOOSTER | **Protect your eyes from your computer**

- Reduce computer eyestrain by taking your eyes away from the computer screen at least once every hour for five minutes. Return a phone call or do some filing. You can also do some eye exercises. Rest your elbows on your desk, palms facing upward. Now bend forward to rest your closed eyes at the base of your palms. Inhale deeply through your nose; hold it for four seconds, and then exhale. Continue for thirty seconds.
- Another exercise involves holding one of your fingers a few inches from your face. Focus on your finger as you slowly move it away, then focus on something in the distance, then bring your focus back to your finger, then watch your finger as you slowly move it toward your face. Then focus on something farther than eight feet away for a few seconds.
- Position your computer monitor so that it's about twenty-eight inches from your eyes—about arm's length. If you feel that you need to be closer to read the type, increase the font size on your display instead. The top of the screen should be at eye level or below so that you look down slightly; having the screen too high or too low can cause neck tension.
- If you wear bifocals or trifocals, you may have a tendency to tilt your head backward to read the screen. Instead, lower the screen a few inches or purchase eyewear specifically designed for computer work. Make sure your eyewear is designed to reduce glare.
- Place your keyboard directly in front of your monitor. If your keyboard is at an angle to the monitor, it tires your eyes by forcing them to focus at varying distances from the screen.
- If you're referring to hard-copy documents, place them on a document holder right next to the screen. This won't force your eyes to readjust constantly.[9]

▲ ▲ ▲

▼ ▼ ▼

▼ ENERGY BANDIT #7 | **Stale air**

Since most of us work indoors, we have to depend on the ventilation system at our place of employment to deliver a steady supply of
fresh air. This might seem a minor concern, since most buildings are
built deliberately to allow as much air in as possible, but in this day
of huge apartment blocks, skyscrapers, and massive call centers, a
good ventilation system—that is, one capable of moving the air
around relatively vigorously—is absolutely necessary for the maintenance of good worker health. Unfortunately, in most structures
ventilation is set up to meet minimum code requirements and to
save money, a consideration that often backfires on the management. The result of poor ventilation can be sick building syndrome
(SBS), in which the low air quality causes increased worker illness
and a concurrent decrease in productivity.[10] Worse, poor ventilation
can result in a buildup of indoor pollution, including molds, which
can have a particularly adverse affect on those with allergies. Poor
ventilation can also spread energy-sapping communicable illnesses
like colds. As the RAND Corporation pointed out in a recent report, taking better care of ventilation "would lead to lower health
care costs, reduced sick leave, and shorter periods of illness-
impaired work performance, resulting in annual economic benefits
for the U.S. in the tens of billions of dollars."[11]

▲ ENERGY BOOSTER | **Insist on proper ventilation**

One of our basic human requirements is a good supply of oxygen,
one of the fuels that power our bodies. If you and your coworkers
seem to be getting sick a lot, or if you're constantly having to fight
off mold, consider checking your building's ventilation system: the
building itself might be sick. While your boss might be a little aggra-

vated if you start poking around in the ventilation ducts (unless, of course, your boss is you), the least you can do is to check out how well the ventilation system is working. This may be as simple as hanging a piece of tinsel on the outflow vent to see how often it runs. Peek inside, if you can, to see if it's looking a little moldy. If you notice any problems, try speaking to your superiors about it, pointing out that good ventilation can increase productivity. If your company doesn't seem to be willing to do the right thing, you can still make your workspace a bright spot in a poorly ventilated office. All it takes is a small, inexpensive fan or electric air purifier to keep you breathing more freely. Another good strategy is to buy plants for your office. Plants like the peace lily or the Chinese evergreen suck toxic chemicals out of the air.

▲ ▲ ▲
▼ ▼ ▼

▼ ENERGY BANDIT #8 | Background noise

From ringing cell phones to cheesy music at the grocery store to all the little whistles and clicks from your computer, your world is rife with background noise. Although reacting to a loud noise is an important survival tool in human evolution, the constant din of today's technology takes a toll on the psyche and therefore your energy.[12] High levels of background noise, such as in an open office space with several cubicles, can compromise the quality of your work. That's especially true for team-oriented work, which is compromised by noise-induced irritability. Background noise can also raise blood pressure, lower performance on complex tasks, cause tension and headaches, and impair concentration.[13] Some people seem to be naturally able to tune out the noise around them, while others experience increased stress and decreased motivation in noisy environments.

Gary Evans and psychologists at Cornell University have found that constant low-level noise in open-style offices increases stress and lowers motivation. Their study assigned forty experienced clerical workers to either a quiet office or one with constant background noise for three hours. The workers in the noisy environment experienced higher stress as measured by their epinephrine levels and made 40 percent fewer attempts to solve a puzzle. Elevated levels of the stress hormone epinephrine can lead to heart disease and musculoskeletal problems.[14]

Researchers at Yale University found that noise stress impairs the brain's cognitive function in the prefrontal cortex. Chronic low-level noise impairs our ability to learn; causes irritability, poor concentration, and fatigue; and compromises work performance. Dr. Alice H. Suter, an audiologist at the National Institute for Occupational Safety and Health, says that noise can cause high blood pressure, peptic ulcers, cardiovascular deaths, stroke, suicidal tendencies, a weakened immune system, learning impairment, and aggression.[15]

▲ ENERGY BOOSTER | **Reduce noise**

Many businesses are aware of the energy-draining effects of noise and install white-noise generators, which broadcast a soothing and (usually) nearly inaudible static that keeps most sound from traveling more than a few dozen feet. If your office doesn't have white-noise generators installed, buffer the outside world with an iPod, Walkman, or MP3 player. Most modern computers can play music files as well; all you need is a good set of earphones. Or you could use a noise-canceling headset while you work. My Bose headset drowns out the sounds of airplane engines; they might be effective against Chatty Cathy's chatter as well. Some people swear by nature-sound machines to help them create their own background noise. When my son James was an infant, he wouldn't sleep at day care unless he had "Birds of Paradise" playing in his ear. His caretakers soon learned to place the little machine in the crib with him, and he slept like they wanted him to: like a baby. I am driven to distraction by these types of machines, but I do well with a soft country-music radio station in the background.

Turn off your computer volume as well. Your psyche is constantly bombarded by all the little clicks and dings your computer makes when it performs the smallest operation—simply decide you don't need it! You need the volume turned up only if you're watching a file with sound, such as a video. You will be *completely amazed* at how much more calmness you exude and how much peace of mind you feel if you try this. Encourage your coworkers to turn off their computer volume as well, to minimize the overall background noise in your office. This is especially helpful if you work in an open-space office with several cubicles.

To further reduce noise in your life, try driving with your radio off. You don't have to be the receptor for all the bad news in the world. That doesn't mean you should be an uncaring person, but there's nothing you can do about a murder that took place yesterday in a different state. It's important to keep abreast of news, but you'd be surprised at how little news you need to keep abreast. Keep the radio on for only ten minutes of your drive, or listen to it every other day. Better yet, put in your favorite CD. Or drive in silence and spend some time thinking some positive thoughts—like reflecting on a recent vacation. Remember the saying "Silence is golden."

▲ ▲ ▲

Sixteen

Relationships

Periphery quiz item #16:
Let's hold hands and sing "Kumbaya"

Do you have friends and family but don't feel close to anyone? Do you have someone to talk with after an argument with your significant other? Even if you're in a relationship and have plenty of acquaintances, you can feel lonely. Research has shown that physical exercise, relaxation, and physical health are positively associated with feelings of well-being, but the variable with the strongest association of all is social support.[1] So if you want to boost feelings of psychological well-being and happiness, have lots of friends. Loneliness undermines health by altering cardiac function and disrupting sleep. The strength of social isolation as a risk factor is comparable to obesity, a sedentary lifestyle, and possibly even smoking. The happiest people surround themselves with family and friends, don't care about keeping up with the Joneses, lose themselves in daily activities, and forgive easily. In this chapter, you'll look at your sources of emotional support, including spouses/partners, children, parents, clubs, friends, volunteer work, and associations. I'll encourage you to reach out to form relationships, make new friends, help others, contribute to your community, and form connections to new sources of joy.

▼ ▼ ▼

▼ ENERGY BANDIT #1 | **Relying on your spouse or significant other as your sole source of friendship**

Just because you're in a romantic relationship doesn't mean that you don't need other friends. I've had a couple of friends with whom I was pretty tight—I thought—who seemed to fall off the face of the planet once they fell in love. Don't become like them. A lack of friends can have damaging repercussions on your mood, your energy level, and even your health. In one study from Carnegie Mellon University in Pittsburgh, freshmen who reported feeling lonely had a weaker immune response to the flu vaccine than those who spent more time among friends.

▲ ENERGY BOOSTER | **Spend time with other friends**

It's important for everyone to have friends outside of marriage and relationships—men and women alike. At the very least, if you and your spouse have an argument, you need to be able to speak to a third party, or simply have a sympathetic shoulder to lean on for a few minutes. If you haven't nurtured any friendships, to whom will you turn for advice or simply to blow off a little steam? Your former best friend whom you haven't contacted in more than a year? Chances are her ear won't be very sympathetic, and her shoulder won't have much room for you to lean on it. Use the following strategies to nurture your friendships:

- If you and your spouse are interested in different activities, take friends along. Your spouse wants to go to the quilting expo, but you'd rather drive a nail through your foot? Encourage her to take a friend instead. And when she groans when you invite her to the speedway race, invite a friend instead, and encourage her to run around with her girlfriends. You don't have to do every single thing together. Remember the old saying "Absence makes the heart grow fonder." You'll have fun stories to share after your outings. Spending a little time apart on a regular basis will renew your relationship instead of letting it grow stale and stagnant.

- Have a women-only party. Women are twice as likely as men to suffer from depression, so it's particularly important for those of the female persuasion to regularly get together with one another.[2] Social gatherings instill a spirit of happiness, joy, and laughter, which can dispel depression. Order party goods from www.femailcreations.com, such as facial and manicure kits, or a game called "Girls Night Out Table Topics." This game includes hilarity-inspiring questions such as "If you woke up to discover that you were a man, what's the first thing you would do?" I have a colleague who used to host an annual women's party. It featured "Trampoline Empowerment" and a swap bag to trade clothing or decorative items, and she made every single guest say something positive about her physical body before stepping foot through the door.

- Schedule a regular girls' night or guys' night out. It can be once a week or once a month. Enjoy teatime, meeting for coffee, or even a beer on the beach. Men may choose to golf, go ice fishing, watch the big game, or smoke cigars while playing poker. Or just get together for coffee or dinner. Encourage your significant other to enjoy time with friends as well.

▲ ▲ ▲

▼ ▼ ▼

▼ ENERGY BANDIT #2 | Being all business at work

Many people mistakenly believe you shouldn't combine work and play. They limit their relationships to "strictly business" at work—and that can be a mistake.

▲ ENERGY BOOSTER | Nurture friendships at your workplace

Managers should pay attention: Tom Rath, author of *Vital Friends: The People You Can't Afford to Live Without* (Gallup Press, August 2006), discovered that people who have good buddies at work are seven times more likely to be engaged in their jobs, and if they have three vital friends at work, they are 96 percent more likely to be satisfied with their lives. So invite a colleague to lunch and get to know him or her. You don't have to be "all work and no play" at the office, or, just like Jack, you will be a dull boy. Be willing to trust a bit and stretch the boundaries if you find someone with whom you connect or seem to have a lot in common. If all goes well, you can start socializing outside the office. If that's just too strange, you can limit your friendship to working hours.

▲ ▲ ▲
▼ ▼ ▼

▼ ENERGY BANDIT #3 | Getting stuck inside the parenting box

Play dates, soccer practice, and rehearsal are great places to meet other people who share the same interests as you—namely, parenting. But this shouldn't be your only social circle. If you're not careful, all your discussions will revolve around your children. While socializing with other parents can be particularly helpful for parents of babies and toddlers, it can develop a life of its own when children are a little older. If all your socializing occurs in the bleachers during practice or with other parent volunteers at your child's school, then your life is not only out of balance, it will disappear completely once your children leave. This can also drain your energy, even if only subconsciously.

▲ ENERGY BOOSTER | **Spend time with people outside your children's circle**

When you became a parent, you did not cease to exist. You are still an individual human being with your own interests, hobbies, and friends. If you don't take time to socialize with other adults in an atmosphere that doesn't revolve around children's activities or making children the centerpiece of conversation, then you're going to wither away. You're not "David's mom," you're "Lori." You're not "David's dad," you're "Robert." If you don't step outside the parenting box on a regular basis, at least once a month, it's tough to recharge your batteries. Stress, fatigue, and even resentment may begin to build up over time, even if you're not consciously aware of it. And an overtaxed parent is a grumpy, impatient parent. Here are some ways to get non-kid time:

- Branch out beyond Gymboree and soccer practice. Although these are great places to meet other parents, you need to enjoy some regular adult time too.
- Make sure you get together with other parents for fun time without the kids. Enjoy attending a house party, concert, or going out to eat together. Split the cost for a babysitter so that all the kids can enjoy playing together while all the parental units get to spend a night on the town. And issue an agreement not to talk about the kids. Get together with

other adults at least once a month. Call some friends, and put a date on the calendar.

- If you can interweave getting together with friends with an activity that's difficult to enjoy with children, you'll get even more energy mileage from it. For example, if you have very small children but love to take daylong hikes, perhaps you and another couple can get a babysitter and take a weekend hiking getaway—complete with a cabin and hot tub.

- Become friends with people who don't have children. This will encourage your conversations to not revolve around kids, kids, kids, which will help your brain function in new and exciting ways. You will be amazed at their energy levels, which will rub off on you. Chances are they'll be involved in many activities since they have more time, and you'll meet even more new people through their different social circles. If they invite you to a dinner party, to a cross-country-skiing outing, or to a fund-raiser, jump at the chance.

▲ ▲ ▲
▼ ▼ ▼

▼ ENERGY BANDIT #4 | **Shyness**

Many people are naturally introverted, and there's nothing wrong with that. It takes all types to make the world go round—from gregarious extroverts to reflective introverts. If it weren't for reflective introverts such as Albert Einstein, the human race wouldn't have made the progress it has. But if you are so painfully shy that you avoid making conversation with others, such as with other people at your table during an awards banquet, then you're hampering your ability to make new friends—and not having friends is detrimental to your mood, energy level, and overall health.

▲ ENERGY BOOSTER | **Uncover the reasons for your shyness and seek to overcome it**

Approximately 5.3 million Americans suffer from social phobia, or social anxiety disorder. This involves an intense, overwhelming fear of everyday social situations; it can even interfere with attending work or school. Beyond deep anxiety, physical symptoms can include blushing, profuse perspiring, trembling, nausea, and difficulty speaking.[3] How did you get so shy? Were your parents overly critical? Did other children or a teacher cruelly insult you? Uprooting the source can help you become more comfortable in social situations. Of course, if your shyness is debilitating, you should seek the assistance of a mental-health practitioner.

Overcoming your shyness doesn't mean that you have to overhaul your basic personality. It just means summoning the courage to introduce yourself at social events instead of hunching over the program in the corner. Take a deep breath and go for it. Everyone else there is a human being, just like you. Nobody's going to grow tentacles and an extra set of eyeballs if you walk up, shake their hand, and say, "Hi, I'm Deb." And if for some strange reason he or she turns out to be a jerk, think of a smooth segue to politely end the conversation, and move on to the next person. This is the only way you're going to find a really great person in life to befriend. Sure, you might have to wade through a room full of boring personalities, but you may find one gem. And you would never have discovered this person if you hadn't jumped in. You'll figure out very quickly whether they're on your wavelength, given their interests and personality. If they are, say something like, "You're really interesting. Do you want to meet for coffee sometime?" It's like the first day of going swimming in the summer. You can either sit there, telling yourself, "The water's too cold," or you can inch your way in. Before you know it, it's time to go, and you haven't even gotten in up to your knees. Or, you can just dive in. It might be a little shocking at first, but you get used to it within a few minutes, and before you know it, you're having fun swimming. And when it's time to leave, you've had a great time.

What do you talk about when you meet new people? That's easy: ask questions. People love to talk about themselves. What are your hobbies? What do you do for a living? Where are you from originally? Do you have children? Eventually the person will ask you questions, and you'll discover whether you have anything in common, such as being addicted to dark chocolate or enjoying hiking.

▲ ▲ ▲
▼ ▼ ▼

▼ ENERGY BANDIT #5 | Isolation from the outside world

Socializing is very important for our health, especially as we age. As a matter of fact, enjoying the company of friends regularly in old age can increase life expectancy even more than visiting regularly with family members. Australian scientists conducted a study of how social, health, and lifestyle factors affected the longevity of more than fifteen hundred people over the age of seventy. The Australian Longitudinal Study of Aging began in 1992; participants' survival rates were recorded during the following decade. They were surveyed about how much personal and telephone contact they enjoyed with friends and relatives. Amazingly, close contact with relatives, including children, had little impact on longevity rates. But participants who enjoyed the strongest network of friends and acquaintances were 22 percent less likely to die during the study period than those with the weakest networks. This proved true even if participants had experienced a stressful life change, such as the death of a spouse or close friends moving away. The study's authors stated that friends have such a positive effect on survival because they're selected, unlike family members; they also stated that friends might more readily encourage one another to look after their health, and that they actively help dispel any feelings of depression or anxiety.[4]

▲ ENERGY BOOSTER | **Stop leaning so heavily on nonhumans for company**

The only time it's acceptable to befriend a nonhuman entity is if you're stranded on a desert island for months on end, as Tom Hanks's character, Chuck Noland, was in the movie *Cast Away*. A volleyball washed up onshore, which he named Wilson, so he would have someone to talk with to keep insanity at bay. If you're an outdoors enthusiast, perhaps you've heard of the Rule of Threes when it comes to survival: humans can survive for three minutes without air, three hours without shelter and protection in freezing weather, three days without water, three weeks without food, and three months without companionship. No matter how shy or Scrooge-like you are, you need relationships with people, not the following non-friends:

- Cigarettes and alcohol are not friends. Don't spend all your time alone with them.
- Your TV, radio, and computer aren't friends. The excessive electromagnetic radiation can disrupt your sleep cycle. Plus, all those ads from pharmaceutical companies will make you think you have every disease imaginable. If your conversations with other human beings revolve around television-show plots, you're spending too much time watching TV.
- Don't use pets as friends. Yes, doggies are "man's best friend" and they provide loads of happiness, silliness, and unconditional love. But pets aren't human. You're doing them, and yourself, a disservice by expecting them to have human qualities. Yes, they can help relieve your stress with their special companionship. But they don't know how to fix that problem

with your annoying boss. You can talk to them, but they don't talk back. Don't become one of those crazy old ladies with eighteen cats.

▲ ▲ ▲
▼ ▼ ▼

▼ ENERGY BANDIT #6 | Not feeling connected to others

Loneliness is far different from aloneness: loneliness is a state of mind, while aloneness is a state of being. Some people can live alone and be perfectly content and happy, while others can be surrounded by family and friends and still feel disconnected. Millions of people suffer from loneliness, which can be caused by divorce, the loss of a loved one, or some other life-altering circumstance. Or perhaps they suffer from low self-esteem or feelings of abandonment, rejection, anxiety, unworthiness, or uselessness. Many times their despair causes them to withdraw from social circles. Temporarily experiencing loneliness from time to time is unavoidable, but chronic loneliness is detrimental to your health. All humans have a fundamental need to belong and to fit in. When that need is not met, you'll feel hopeless and lack the energy to extend yourself to others.

▲ ENERGY BOOSTER | Get plugged in with others of similar likes

Loneliness feeds on loneliness. The more a person experiences feelings of despair, the harder it is to break from that cycle. But loneliness doesn't have to be a way of life. As with changing any behavior pattern, it takes effort and commitment to begin to move in a more positive direction. You must aggressively attack your sense of feeling disconnected. If you do not aggressively attack loneliness, you run the risk of getting trapped in chronic desolation. You might start to condemn yourself to solitary confinement, either mentally, physically, or both. Use these tactics to get connected to others:

- Become active in a local club that shares your interests. My church has a program called "After 49ers" for people, well, older than forty-nine. They meet monthly, go on tours, have guest speakers, put on holiday bazaars, and otherwise have a great time together. This is a wonderful way for people of the same age to meet others who enjoy the same pastimes. And you never know—you may even see someone there you know, but you had no idea they shared your interest. What are your hobbies? Writing poetry? Photography? Hiking? Playing guitar? Figure out what you love, or get involved in something new. Increase your enjoyment of your favorite activities by sharing them with those who are like-minded.

- Look through your local newspapers' event calendars to find activities that match your interests. You can also browse flyers posted at your local library or post office, listen to your local radio station's calendar of events, or view calendars on Web sites of local TV stations. You'll find poetry readings, open-microphone nights, group hikes, and free lectures galore.

- Find a local organization of your political persuasion. These organizations' activities go beyond canvassing during election time; they also have summer cookouts just for fun and camaraderie.

- If there are no clubs or events in your area that match your interests, create your own. Put an ad in the local paper, post some flyers at the library and post office, and post it on a local e-mail ListServ.

- Do you want to hone your public-speaking skills? Try Toastmasters. If you're already speaking twenty or more times a year, you're eligible to join my professional association, the National Speakers Association (www.nsaspeaker.org). The relationships I've built over the years are an invaluable source of friendship and advice. Going to the national conventions and educational forums rejuvenates and inspires me for the next few months.

- Are you a veteran? Join the local VFW or American Legion.

▲ ▲ ▲
▼ ▼ ▼

▼ ENERGY BANDIT #7 | Overscheduling your children

Alvin Rosenfeld, M.D., author of *The Over-Scheduled Child: Avoiding the Hyper-Parenting Trap*, says today's parents feel more societal and parental peer pressure to provide their children with more opportunities. William Doherty, professor of family social science at the University of Minnesota and author of *Take Back Your Kids*, says today's parents tend to perceive their children as "bundles of creative potential." Therefore, they enroll their children in numerous activities to maximize that potential. No more time for riding bikes around the neighborhood, playing tag, or playing kick the can.[5]

▲ ENERGY BOOSTER | Spend plenty of quality time with your children

Family dinnertime is usually the first thing to go. According to the Food Marketing Institute, only 40 percent of American families eat dinner together, yet just a generation ago, 80 percent of families enjoyed the evening meal together. Professor Doherty says that dinnertime makes children feel that their parents are interested in them. Also, when family members don't take the time to enjoy a proper dinner, they fall prey to the garbage in, garbage out cycle: junk food, highly processed foods, and fast food, which are giant energy drains.[6]

Children need structure, but they—and you—don't need to be exhausted. Look at the big picture with all your children's schedules when deciding whether to allow them to undertake a particular extracurricular activity. Your children should be allowed to pursue their interests, but it shouldn't cross the line into being overscheduled. If your family can eat dinner together only three times a week or less and the children are consistently up past their bedtime, chances are they are overscheduled. Your children don't *want* all that activity—they just want YOU. Spending time with your children makes them feel loved and important, increasing their self-esteem.

Set some reasonable rules. My favorite with my kids is "One season, one sport." Tell your child he/she must choose only one sport to focus on each season. For example, if playing on both volleyball and basketball teams occurs in the same season, pick one over the other. If your child really enjoys soccer but also wants to ride horses, take a hiatus from riding during the spring soccer season. Then ride during the summer until soccer begins again in the fall. When it's too cold to play soccer or ride horses, take a few months of swimming lessons at an indoor pool.

▲ ▲ ▲
▼ ▼ ▼

▼ ENERGY BANDIT #8 | **Stressful relationships**

You might not like the people you work with. Your boss might annoy you: that's life. But that does not mean that you should force yourself to stick with a job where you have an abusive boss or the workplace is continually wrought with chronic dysfunctional politics. Sometimes things can't be worked out, and it makes the most sense to leave. But leaving a stressful relationship isn't always possible. You can't escape your immediate family members. You can't fire them and hire new ones. You're stuck with your parents, and you're stuck with your kids. Sure, the kids will move out of the house someday, but that doesn't help you right now. And you can elect to visit your parents only a few times a year, but they're still your parents no matter how you slice it.

▲ ENERGY BOOSTER | Work through relationship problems

For some reason, many of us equate not saying anything at all with being nice. But when you don't speak up, all that happens is that it festers inside you and preoccupies your mind with negativity. You may even become subconsciously passive-aggressive. This drains not only your energy but that of everyone around you. Your boss and teenager deserve special mention:

- If the boss asks you for feedback about his or her performance, offer it. Don't zip your lip in hopes of a better chance for a raise or promotion. "I feel it's not the most efficient use of our time to have a twenty-minute meeting every time you need to add something to my to-do list. If the explanation or instructions don't require a lot of detail, perhaps you could send me a thirty-second e-mail. Then I would have more time to accomplish more projects faster. Would that work for you?" But don't wait for someone to ask for feedback. If it's nagging at you, get it off your chest. "You need to remember to always put your dishes in the dishwasher."
- Keep your teenagers' angst in perspective. As a parent, you have to let some of their bizarre behavior slip past you. If you start disciplining every single instance, they'll find more dangerous ways to rebel—such as drinking and driving. However, know where to draw the line. Explain to them that while they may be upset with you right now, they do have to treat you with at least the same consideration that they would offer a grocery-store cashier. Politely remind them to watch

their tone of voice, the evil eye, or the big sighs. If they don't follow the rules, dole out a punishment with a lot of "ouch" value, such as taking away the iPod or laptop for the rest of the day. They may seethe even more in the confines of their bedroom after slamming the door, but it's your job to teach them that they should treat others with basic courtesy. It's good practice for when they'll have to deal with quirky bosses as an adult.

▲ ▲ ▲

Seventeen

Stress

Your body takes a beating from chronic stress in the form of minor problems such as sweaty palms, headaches, backaches, fatigue, and memory loss—not to mention major problems such as heart disease, depression, and hypertension. The body produces too many steroids when it's under stress, which can upset the acid balance of the stomach, causing pain and ulcers. Charles Wood, a professor of physiology at the University of Florida College of Medicine, says, "Steroids can also depress the immune system, which may be why chronically tense people are prone to colds and other illnesses." In fact, the physical effects of stress are so wide-ranging and common that some experts estimate that almost half of all doctor visits are stress-related. If you experience the stress response often enough, your body has to store more fat for these occasions. Cortisol increases fat deposits most frequently in the belly—meaning stress can literally make you fat. People with high stress levels are more likely to have heart attacks and strokes, respond less well to flu vaccines, and catch colds more easily than those with low levels of work or interpersonal stress. I'll show you how to shift your perception and the impact of those situations. You'll stop trying to control the uncontrollable and instead focus on what you can control—yourself and your reactions.

▼ ▼ ▼

▼ ENERGY BANDIT #1 | High anxiety levels

According to a study reported in the May 2001 issue of the *American Journal of Psychiatry*, the monthly scientific journal of the American Psychiatric Association, absenteeism due to health problems was twice as high for employees with depressive symptoms as those without depressive symptoms. The study also revealed that the likelihood of decreased performance on the job is seven times higher for depressed employees.

▲ ENERGY BOOSTER | Take psychological steps to reduce your anxiety level

To keep depression from making you sick and sapping your energy, stress management can be a key part of your treatment plan. Here are a few things you can try:

- Pray or meditate. Harold Koenig, a psychiatrist at Duke University Medical Center in Durham, North Carolina, says that twenty minutes of prayer or meditation might lower blood pressure, reduce anxiety, cut stress levels, and perhaps even help people live longer.[1]
- Use positive imagery to help elevate your mood and inspire you.
- See a psychologist or participate in a company-sponsored employee assistance program (EAP) if you find stress control hard to practice on your own. Licensed professionals can help you maintain good emotional health by treating depression, teaching you anger-management techniques, or finding ways to relax.
- Forgive someone. If you're harboring a grudge against some-

one, you'll want to clean your emotional slate. Forgiveness is not a sign of weakness; it's a sign of strength. Reliving a bad experience in your mind or experiencing bitter feelings every day can really eat at you. Resolve to stop wasting energy on negative thoughts that diminish your ability to put energy into new and exciting endeavors. Visit www.forgiving.org for advice on how to let go of grudges.

▲ ▲ ▲
▼ ▼ ▼

▼ ENERGY BANDIT #2 | Not practicing good stress-management techniques

You can't just sit back and expect your high stress levels to subside. You have to *do* something about them. When something stressful happens to you, you've got two choices: you can let it get to you and drain your energy, or you can take steps to distract yourself. I'm not talking about denial, that handy psychological prop that lets you ignore bad things. Internalizing all the uncontrollable aspects of your life will just give you an ulcer.

▲ ENERGY BOOSTER | Actively counter stress

In addition to working on the emotional component of stress, you can physically DO some things to alleviate it:

- Get a massage. An increasing number of research studies show that massage reduces heart rate, lowers blood pressure, increases blood circulation and lymph flow, relaxes muscles, improves range of motion, and increases endorphins (enhancing medical treatment). At the Touch Research Institute at the University of Miami School of Medicine, researchers have found that massage is helpful in decreasing blood pressure in people with hypertension, alleviating pain in migraine and fibromyalgia sufferers, enhancing immune function, and improving alertness and performance in office workers. Many of these effects appear to be mediated by decreased stress hormones after massage.[2]

- Listen to music. Carl Charnetski, Ph.D., a psychology professor at Wilkes University in Wilkes-Barre, Pennsylvania, conducted several studies on how music raises IgA levels, your body's natural defense in fighting germs, especially during times of stress. After listening to jazz music for half an hour, newspaper reporters who were on deadline had increased IgA levels, which continued to rise for at least thirty minutes after the music stopped playing.[3] So break out your iPod, MP3 player, or CD player, and your body will thank you with improved immunity, fewer illnesses, and lower stress—a triple-whammy energy booster.

- Cry. Rather than being a sign of weakness, weeping can be an effective stress-reduction method. Remember all those times you were emotionally distraught, and people told you to "Let it all out," or "You'll feel better after a good cry"? Well, they were right. Crying is a visceral, sudden release of built-up tension that helps you get through an emotional reaction to some event or sequence of events. There's even a complementary (i.e., alternative) therapeutic stress-reduction method called "bioenergetics" that encourages crying (along with shouting, biofeedback, and herbal treatments).[4]

▲ ▲ ▲

▼ ▼ ▼

▼ ENERGY BANDIT #3 | Uncontrollable situations

You can decide what to eat, what to wear, and what kind of car to drive. But you can't control a traffic jam, your company's direction, or Mother Nature. How much energy do you devote to things you can't control? We all face annoying situations like waiting in long lines and having to deal with irritating coworkers. No matter how competent you are, and no matter how long or how hard you work, you can't control everything. The weather's going to change against your will, and all those other people out there have their own agendas to follow.

▲ ENERGY BOOSTER | Seize control in small ways

Identify the things you can and can't control in your daily life. Once you've done this, you can work on the things you have some control over, and let the rest go. Remember the old Serenity Prayer, the staple of most 12-step programs? It goes something like this: "God, grant me the serenity to accept the things I cannot change, the courage to change those that I can, and the wisdom to know the difference." While it sounds a bit trite to some of us, it's that way because it's so true.

If you're feeling powerless, whatever you do, don't just sit there and let it overwhelm you—or your energy and motivation will drain away, and you'll just sit wringing your hands. You can't eliminate the stress in your life, but you can learn to take control in small ways. What does this mean for you? That you should prove to yourself that you *are* in control, even if that proof comes only from small actions: finishing an item on your to-do list, practicing positive thinking, fixing the broken handle on the toilet, managing to lose a pound or two, or learning a new language. Although much of our stress comes from outside, some of it is self-inflicted. Other small ways to seize control may simply involve attitude adjustments:

- Don't let others get your goat. If you're doing the best you can but there's absolutely nothing you can do to make a specific person happy, don't let it get to you. This includes bosses, teachers, and significant others. While it's true that these people may be able to punish you for not meeting their standards, you can't let that stop you from being in control of your own fate. As the singer Ricky Nelson once pointed out, "You can't please everyone, so you've got to please yourself."
- Break loose from perfectionism. Instead of worrying about doing everything just right, just get things done as best as you can.
- Make decisions and let them go. Don't agonize over a choice once it's done. It's a fact that you're going to make mistakes now and then; it's what separates humans from the divine. Unless you're a doctor or a military officer, it's doubtful that most of your decisions will be life-or-death ones.

▲ ▲ ▲
▼ ▼ ▼

▼ ENERGY BANDIT #4 | Job stress

People in jobs with high work demands, low levels of job control, and little workplace social support are more likely to suffer poor health—and see their energy decline—than people in more flexible jobs with reasonable demands and social support. Stress on the job can not only eat up your energy and send you spiraling down into depression, but it can also make you become a not-so-nice person whom no one wants to be around. It all starts to emerge in your emotions and behavior—but it can then turn into the physical symptoms I've already mentioned. Following are typical enablers of job stress:

- Feelings of powerlessness or lack of control
- Having to work straight through lunch and breaks, either from personal choice or by direct order
- Uncertainty about job security
- Job dissatisfaction
- Work overload
- Work *under*load
- Poor scheduling
- Unclear demands
- Physical conditions

Whatever the causes of job-related stress, the results are many and obvious, and can all contribute to a loss of personal energy in the workplace, which can lead to other effects:

- Pessimism
- Dissatisfaction
- Lack of concentration
- Decreased motivation
- Accidents
- Absenteeism
- Poor health[5]

Clearly it's in your company's best interests to fix the problems that are causing your job stress to manifest in the above symptoms, but you can't expect every company's management team to be that enlightened—or even to notice that there's something wrong. Therefore, you've got to take matters into your own hands and develop your own strategies to stay sane.

▲ ENERGY BOOSTER | Turn off work when you're on personal time

It can be hard for any of us, especially the self-employed, to follow this suggestion. The advent of efficient, easy-to-use mobile devices has caused the boundaries between work time and home time to shift and become extremely nebulous; it's too easy to check your e-mail or call someone across the continent, even when you're supposed to be at home enjoying your leisure time. This kind of "work-extending technology" is a dual-edged sword, in that it allows us to be productive outside normal working hours, but it cuts into the time we need for recharging our batteries, which ultimately cuts into our productivity.[6] Your boss may not want to hear it, but it's absolutely necessary to separate your personal and work time if you want to maintain any enthusiasm for the job you're doing. The alternative is job burnout, and the loss of effective productivity that comes with it. If at all possible, let your workday end when you leave your office.

▲ ▲ ▲
▼ ▼ ▼

▼ ENERGY BANDIT #5 | Not using all the benefits to which you're entitled

We may not have it as good as our parents did when it comes to our employers taking care of us—and we certainly don't have it as good as the Europeans—but most of us still have decent benefits, many of which we don't use.

▲ ENERGY BOOSTER | Take full advantage of company-sponsored benefit plans

Benefits vary, of course, but some of the more common are as follows:

- Regular breaks. By law, anyone who works more than six hours a day should get two fifteen-minute breaks and at least a half hour for lunch. These breaks don't exist just so you can be lazy, although some managers certainly seem to think that's the case. The whole point of breaks is to get you away from your task, if only for a few minutes, so you can stretch your mental and physical muscles and get a little rest. Focusing too tightly on something for too long can cause you to lose your mental edge, even if your focus remains sharp.
- Flex time. Some companies allow employees to work four ten-hour days and take a full Friday off, or work four nine-hour days and leave at noon on Friday. This is an excellent way to recharge your batteries or get some errands done.
- Flexible scheduling. Some companies may allow you to come in at a different hour than the traditional 8:00 or 9:00 AM, as long as you get in your full forty hours per week. This is another way to organize your work schedule so it's more advantageous to you.
- Floating holidays. Some companies provide a day off on your birthday, or possibly any other day you choose. Take advantage of these, so you don't get too overwhelmed.
- Job sharing. This is regular part-time work in which two people voluntarily share the responsibilities of one full-time, salaried position with benefits.
- Sabbatical. Some companies will allow you to take several months off after every five years of work or a year off after twenty. This can be paid or unpaid but guarantees your job when you return.

- Sick days. If you're sick, be sick. Most companies prefer that you stay at home instead of potentially infecting the entire office with the cold or flu (a phenomenon called "presenteeism," which most of us have experienced). It's not unheard of to use a sick day as a "mental health" day, either, when the workaday world of the office just gets to be too much.
- Telecommuting. Modern technology makes it simple for those of us with jobs in the technology sector to telecommute, assuming we have an Internet connection and a phone. Ask for permission to telecommute, if it's a benefit your company offers. On high-stress days, or when you just can't handle the traffic without going nuts, stay at home and work.
- Take a vacation. Although Americans are woefully underprovided with vacations compared to most Europeans, most of us can count on two to three weeks of paid vacation a year. Try to take every minute you can, in order to help you revitalize yourself and stay fresh.

▼ ENERGY BANDIT #6 | You create crisis on purpose

The adrenaline rush you experience when stressed can be quite addictive. Some people like it and cause it to happen so they can experience it—like a drug. Adrenaline junkies get "high" on the rush. They don't feel they're really living unless they're stressed out—physically, mentally, emotionally, or all of the above. They find reasons to get worked up so that they can get a fix of adrenaline, which can be just as addictive as cocaine or any other narcotic. Basically, you're getting high off naturally produced endorphins, adrenaline, cortisol, and corticosteroids.[7] The ultimate result of an adrenaline rush is a subsequent energy crash, and the low is probably worse than any high you can experience.

▲ ENERGY BOOSTER | **Avoid crisis by working ahead of deadlines**

Poor planning, like procrastination, can end up forcing you to do everything at the last minute, which just ratchets up the stress and adds to the difficulty of getting it done. To reduce time spent on crisis management, spend time doing long-term, proactive, important activities, rather than always responding to the urgent. Don't facilitate crisis in your life by procrastinating on tasks until they become urgent. You could do the following in advance:

- Wrap the present days *before* the birthday party (not in the car on the way).
- Refill your prescription several pills *before* you take the last pill (not after you've run out of them, forcing you to wait at the pharmacy thirty minutes before work).
- Find your tax receipts a month *before* taxes are due (not when you're forced to file an extension).
- Stock up on stamps *before* they're gone (and you have to stand in a one-hour line during lunch to mail a single bill).
- Take your printer in for maintenance *before* it breaks down (and you're forced to purchase another so you can get a mailing out while that one is in the shop).

You will be amazed at the level of calm you experience when you do things before they are due or before you need them. Over a period of weeks and months, if you spend ten minutes more a day (building to thirty and sixty minutes more every day) doing activities before they're required, soon you'll have shifted your time wisely. Yes, you're still doing the same activities, but you're no longer doing them under deadlines. The biggest bonus, however, will be the amazing sense of tranquillity you feel by dealing only with life's true emergencies. Ask yourself: what ideas, projects, and programs—if implemented now or in the near future—would significantly impact the profitability or productivity of your staff or your organization?

▲ ▲ ▲
▼ ▼ ▼

▼ ENERGY BANDIT #7 | A type A personality

Let's face it: some people are just more laid back than others. They can handle everyday stresses better than most, without the hormonal and psychological changes that cause the less sanguine among us to lose or misdirect our personal energy. If you're that way yourself, congratulations—you're less likely to get an ulcer than the rest of us. If you're not, you may be a type A personality, which can have effects on your body far beyond energy drain.

Type A personalities tend to be competitive, aggressive, dominant, ambitious, acquisitive, self-driven, hardworking—does this all sound familiar? Some of these traits may have helped you succeed in the business world. In type A personalities, however, these traits are coupled with less-positive traits like impatience, chronic self-criticism, hostility, and a deep-seated insecurity (no matter how much self-assurance the person may exude). There's a sense of urgency in everything they do, something that physicians Meyer Friedman and Ray Rosenman call "hurry sickness."

▲ ENERGY BOOSTER | Don't accept a type A personality as "just the way I am"

Where does a type A personality come from? Though some type A personalities are born, most seem to be made. Even if you were a lovable, laid-back person before your latest promotion, you might find yourself changing after having had enormous amounts of new responsibility dumped upon you. The following traits are common to type A personalities:[8]

- Finishing sentences quickly
- Heavily accenting key words in your speech
- Moving, walking, and eating rapidly
- Open irritation at the rate at which events normally occur
- A tendency to want to hurry the speech of others
- Extreme irritation at everyday delays
- Constant multitasking
- Feelings of guilt when relaxing more than a few hours
- Being bothered watching someone do something when you know you can do it faster
- Pride in numbers: how much you make, how much you spend, how much you can get done in a set amount of time

Just because you display a few of these symptoms doesn't mean you're a type A personality. However, if many or all of them do apply, then sit down: I've got some bad news for you. Type A personalities experience not just energy drain but significant stress- and circulatory-related illnesses much more often than other people. These include heart attacks, strokes, high blood pressure, aneurysms—you name it.

You can take steps to change. There are plenty of ways to help yourself, primarily by relaxing on a regular basis, and taking away some of the stressors that can cause an everyday Joe to transform into a type A ogre.

▲ ▲ ▲

▼ ▼ ▼

Things seem to go wrong when you're in a hurry: you get caught in traffic, you have to wait for someone to get off a conference call, you have to stand in a line, you have to wait for service in a store or a restaurant, and so forth.

▲ ENERGY BOOSTER | **Find something to do that will occupy your mind**

It's better to be creative and productive than to stew because you can't get anything done. Distract yourself in some way:

- I like to pull out my Treo and catch up on my e-mail. Or I check voice mail and return calls. You could have a report with you to edit, thank-you notes to write, or planning for the rest of the month. You may be able to do this only in fits and starts, but it's amazing how much faster it makes the time go—and it can make you feel a lot better to get something done during what would otherwise be wasted downtime.
- Walk away from the problem. This works best with people situations; you certainly don't want to walk away from a traffic jam. Michael Douglas tried that in the movie *Falling Down,* and ended up coming unglued emotionally and psychologically. It's not necessary to be rude; just extricate yourself as soon as possible, before all your personal energy is used up or soured by stress and worry. Say something like, "Let's take a break now and revisit this topic when we can take a more productive approach."
- Endure it. If it's a people situation you can't easily walk away

from (such as a problem with your boss), endure it as best as you can and get away as soon as possible.

- Distract yourself. If you're stuck in traffic, don't stew in your own juice. Make sure your air conditioner is working, crank up the radio to your favorite music, and sing as loudly as you must to keep from exploding. So what if people see you singing? They'll probably think you're using Bluetooth to talk on your cell phone.

- Focus your mind. If you're stuck in a line at the post office, DMV, bank, or wherever, make sure you have something to read. It can be a trashy romance novel, a college text, a corporate report, a magazine, or anything else, as long as it's there. Once again, the idea is to keep from going crazy while you wait.

▲ ▲ ▲

Eighteen

Technology

Periphery quiz item #18:
The Treo: me, you, and your handheld

I've given presentations on productivity since 1992. Especially over the last ten years, I've noticed a marked difference in the feelings of overwork in my audiences. I attribute much of this to the increased use of technology such as cell phones, BlackBerries, beepers, e-mail, and computers. Desktop alerts, instant messages, and dings control our time and tell us what to do. Then we go home, and television, MP3 players, the Internet, computer games, handheld Game Boys, Xbox gaming systems, DVD players, cell phones, and iPods continue to dominate our time. Even the labor-saving devices in our homes have eliminated much of the work involved in doing household chores.

In this chapter, you'll determine if blurring the boundaries of your work and home has made you feel more overworked and less energized. I'll discuss how to break free from technology, turn it off regularly, stop letting it control you, and unplug in ways that boost your energy. We'll chat about habits around usage, addictions to the "Crackberry," and how to gain control.

▾ ▾ ▾

Associating with televisions and computers, rather than people

It isn't natural to stare at a screen (computer, Gameboy, television) for hours on end, day after day, with no interaction with other people. Yet this is precisely what many people do. The subsequent feelings of social isolation and depression can be quite damaging to your energy level.

▲ ENERGY BOOSTER | **Plan your screen time and stick to it**

When I was a child, I was allowed to watch two hours of television each week. When the Sunday TV guide came in the newspaper, I would plan my shows for the week (usually *Little House on the Prairie* and *The Wonderful World of Disney*). I think that because I didn't watch much television as a child, I don't watch it as an adult. When John and I first got married, I thought he watched an inordinate amount of television. For my birthday present one year, I asked him to go on a TV diet, and he obliged by turning off the cable for one month. Today he will tell you it was one of the best decisions he's ever made. He broke his addiction to TV and created time to dedicate to his hobbies and working out.

Did I say "addiction"? How many hours would someone have to devote to gambling or drinking before it could be labeled as an addiction? During the 2004 to 2005 television season (September 20, 2004, to September 18, 2005), the typical American *household* watched television for a whopping eight hours and eleven minutes every day. During the same season, the average *American* actively watched television for four hours and thirty-two minutes a day. That's 12.5 percent higher than one decade earlier, and the highest since Nielson Media Research began charting television usage in the 1950s.[1] When you look at these numbers, you'll see a four-hour gap between having the television *on* and actually *watching* it. If you're not actively watching it, the television is simply background noise (which, as we've seen, can be an energy drain in and of itself).

Watching television is also linked to obesity in both children and adults. Researchers at the Johns Hopkins University School of Medicine, in conjunction with experts from the Centers for Disease Control and the National Institutes of Health, found that children's weight increases in proportion to the number of hours that they watch television every day.[2] No wonder the Office of the Surgeon General says obesity has more than doubled since 1980. A Harvard School of Public Health study published in *The Journal of the American Medical Association* followed more than fifty thousand women for six years and found that for every two hours spent watching television daily, obesity went up by 23 percent and the risk for type 2 diabetes jumped by 14 percent.

So decide to reduce tube time. If you reduced your television time by only five hours a week, you'd gain almost eleven days a year. What could you do with eleven days a year? Spend more time with someone you love? Think of all the wonderful things you could achieve if you spent less time watching television. You could spend the time you normally watch television on your favorite leisure activity, playing with the kids, or accomplishing items on your to-do list. Or writing that novel you've been putting off.

I'm not suggesting you rid yourself of *all* television, just think carefully the next time you reach for the remote. If you feel particularly rested, motivated, educated, or inspired after watching a particular show, fine. But don't keep it on passively in the background. Pick a show and turn it on and off purposefully. Sensible limits may relieve guilt from overindulging, while freeing up time for more worthwhile pursuits. Use these ideas to help you cut back:

- Watch only a select handful of favorite shows a week. Then promptly turn off the TV when each show ends so it doesn't cross the line into becoming background noise.
- Shut off the TV at least a half hour before bedtime, preferably one hour, to allow your already relaxed brain to integrate rapid-fire images; this will improve the quality of your sleep and therefore boost your energy level.
- TiVo or record shows to DVD. Then you can skip the commercials and watch whenever you'd like. Don't stay up until eleven o'clock waiting for your favorite late-night show to come on.

▲ ▲ ▲
▼ ▼ ▼

▼ ENERGY BANDIT #2 | **Letting technology suck up your free time**

How many hours a day do you spend watching television, surfing the Internet, playing video games, and doing e-mail? And how has all of this affected your private time and your personal life? Do you ever log into your office e-mail at night via personal computer for just one more peek, instead of spending time with your family?

▲ ENERGY BOOSTER | **Put your life first**

Technology exists to simplify your life, not to complicate it. It's up to you to keep it in check, or it can literally eat up all your time. Keep technology from interfering with your private life:

- Turn all electronic devices off one hour before bedtime, so you can quiet your mind. This includes laptops, computers, iPods, Gameboys, PlayStations, BlackBerries, cell phones, regular phones, and the television. Have a nice cup of hot tea. Gaze into space. Stretch. Read. Meditate. Spend time with your children. You can't attempt to sleep with all those to-dos and leftover conversations running around in your mind.

- Limit your Web surfing. Ever sit down to look something up on the Web and later look up at the clock, only to discover that you just spent two hours surfing in cyberspace? Mindlessly surfing the Web not only wastes time but also brings you lots of information that is of little use to you. Go to the Web with a specific purpose in mind, focus on the task, and skip the rest.

- Refuse to let the computer and cell phone impede your interaction with other human beings. If you have children, have you ever noticed how you must ask them repeatedly to turn their eyes from the computer screen and truly listen to what you are saying? Have you ever kept your back turned to a coworker while you continued to work on your computer screen? Have you ever noticed your coworkers doing that to you? Computer screens are just as addictive as television screens. Unlock your gaze from the computer monitor so that you can clearly communicate with others, which will save time and energy from rework in the long run. Have you ever seen the funny sight of two friends at a restaurant together, both of whom are talking on their cell phones? Also, don't allow other members of your family—most notably teenagers—to e-mail or call you from another room in your very own home.

▲ ▲ ▲
▼ ▼ ▼

▼ ENERGY BANDIT #3 | **Electronic buildup**

Your voice mailbox is so full that callers receive a message stating there's no more room. Your e-mail in-box is so full of messages that a very important and time-sensitive communication fell through the cracks, straining a friend's or client's trust in you. You have only three or four subfolders in your computer document files, and you have a tendency to save most documents in your main folder; it usually takes you at least five minutes to find a particular document.

Electronic disorganization can be just as energy- and time-sapping as physical disorganization. Not immediately deleting old or irrelevant messages can make your life seem clogged and render you sluggish, lethargic, and overwhelmed. As with a to-do list, the idea is to flow, not to dam. Not organizing your e-mails or your computer files in a streamlined fashion eats up your time, depleting your energy.

▲ ENERGY BOOSTER | Keep your e-mail in-box empty

Slash through the electronic detritus to maximize your efficiency and therefore your energy level:

- Install a powerful spam blocker on your computer. Federal laws regarding spam are weak at best, so it's not going away anytime soon. My e-mail is filtered both server-side by my ISP and on my computer.
- Create folders in your e-mail program. Set a few parameters in your program so that different messages from different categories are automatically sent to a particular folder (e.g., in Outlook, these are called "Rules"). For example, you could have a personal folder, a professional folder, and a parenting folder. We all have at least one friend who for some reason feels compelled to forward each and every corny message he or she receives. There's no reason that detritus has to crowd your main in-box. It can go straight to your personal folder. Ditto for parenting e-mail groups for your child's school.
- Delete, delete, delete. Don't even look at those corny e-mails your friend always forwards. Don't even look at parenting

e-mails that don't concern you. Maybe it's a message about an issue you care about, but if you haven't looked at it in a week, delete it. When you're finished tending to a message in your main in-box, delete it. Delete messages in your deleted-items folder that you don't need to keep permanently, and empty your trash folder at least once a week.

- Keep your in-box thinned. The moment you've finished tending to a message in your main in-box, get rid of it. Get it out of your sight either by filing it in a folder, converting it to a task for follow-up, or deleting it. Keep your in-box so thinned out that the list of messages never extends below the bottom of the window. This will decrease your stress level and keep your energy flowing at its best. Out with the old, and in with the new.

▲ ▲ ▲
▼ ▼ ▼

▼ ENERGY BANDIT #4 | Poor computer organization

What happened to the paperless office? We generate more paper now than we ever did before the advent of the computer! A computer's hard drive can get just as cluttered as any other part of the office. With seemingly limitless storage capacity, it's easy to create piles of files on your computer.

▲ ENERGY BOOSTER | Get organized

- Delete old files on your computer that you don't use regularly or won't need again. Don't keep different file formats of the same document. For example, if you're a graphic designer, you don't need to keep the Adobe Illustrator and the PDF versions of a newsletter you designed. Just keep the original

Illustrator version; you can create another PDF in just a couple of minutes if for some reason you need to down the road. If you have cyclical work, delete the prior files. For example, if you're a managing editor of a quarterly journal, there's no reason to keep each issue's edited documents; just keep them until the next round of articles comes in, then delete all of them. The final version of the articles is in the published version of the journal, and that's all you need. Hone all your electronic documents down to the bare minimum. Not only will this boost your energy, but it will also help your computer continue to run efficiently and quickly. Empty your recycle bin or deleted items regularly to reclaim disk space.

- Create several subfolders. And create subfolders within subfolders. Virtual organization is just as important and time-saving as physical organization. Let's say you're an accountant, and you have a home-based office. You have ten clients. Create a folder for your business. Then create ten subfolders, one for each client. Within each client's folder, create a folder for each category of work performed; for example, monthly financial statements, payroll, ledger, taxes. Each document within each work-category folder should include a date in the file name, with at least the relevant year. You may also need the month and day, depending on your type of work. Then *whip, bang, boom*—you find everything you need in a snap, which preserves your efficient functioning level. And of course, being an accountant, you would be familiar with IRS regulations about how long to keep files, and the first week of every year you would delete all records from all file folders that are no longer necessary to keep.

- Create naming conventions for your files. Now that you've located the correct subfolder, you have to give it a name that will make it easy to find later. I save contracts in the format YYMMDD CLIENT PROGRAM, so that they are in chronological order when I view them.

- Use descriptive titles. When I first started using computers, they were all DOS-based (now I'm showing my age). I used to have to name files with eight letters. Thank heavens for Windows! Now we have a 255-character capability for file names, so go ahead and make the name as long as you want. The bigger the name, the more likely you will be able to find it again using a keyword search. Ask yourself, "If I want this file again, what words or phrases would I think of first?"

▲ ▲ ▲
▼ ▼ ▼

▼ ENERGY BANDIT #5 | **Leaving electronic devices on all the time**

Cell phones, e-mail, BlackBerries, instant messaging—all these technological inventions are designed to make our lives easier. But we have to control them, not vice versa. We never turn off our cell phones, so we never have a break, whether we're driving, at the grocery, or on vacation. What began as efficient multitasking has morphed into never having a peaceful moment to ourselves during the course of a day. We can too easily get pulled into endless rounds of instant messaging—before we know it, an hour has elapsed, and our daily to-do list has become backlogged. We look at the messages in our in-box over and over, trying to remind ourselves about particular action items and how we will accomplish them.

▲ ENERGY BOOSTER | **Turn off your technology when you're on personal time**

When you take a break today, go for a ten-minute walk outdoors—and leave your cell phone in the office. Never turning off the cell phone decreases your productivity during work hours because you constantly have to react to a ringing phone. Unless your job requires you to be "on call," don't leave it on all day. Never turning it off during personal time invades your privacy, never giving you a moment to yourself to rejuvenate your energy levels. If your cell phone is primarily for personal use, turn it off at work. If it's primarily for professional use, turn it off at home. Seriously consider whether you want to talk on your cell phone while driving. The Human Factors and Ergonomics Society reported that using cell phones while driving causes 2,600 deaths and 330,000 injuries in the United States every year. A study published by the society in 2001 found that drivers using cell phones were 18 percent slower to react to brake lights, and took 17 percent longer to regain speed after braking, causing traffic jams. The same holds true for hands-free headsets, because the driver is simply distracted by the conversation. As a matter of fact, drivers talking on cell phones are more impaired than drunk drivers with a blood-alcohol content of 0.08 percent—they have a slower reaction time of several seconds, rather than a fraction of a second. That translates to stopping distances increased by entire car lengths.[3]

Leave your computer off all weekend, or, at the very least, one entire day of the weekend. Resist the urge to sneak back into your office while your family hangs out elsewhere in the house. If you stay connected to your e-mail and cell phone all weekend, you will go to bed physically and mentally exhausted on Sunday night. Instead of starting the week recharged, alert, and efficient, you will be sluggish on Monday morning.

▲ ▲ ▲
▼ ▼ ▼

▼ ENERGY BANDIT #6 | **Technological distractions**

Everyone has had the experience of driving down the road approaching a red light. Let's say two of the three lanes are occupied by other cars. So of course you switch lanes to position yourself in the empty lane—the "pole position." As you slow down and prepare to stop, the light suddenly turns green. Because you are still rolling, instead of stopping you punch the accelerator and zoom past the other two cars. Since they both had to start from a dead stop, you're almost to the next light before they're barely through the intersection. That's inertia. It's the ability to move forward easily when you already have speed. When you have to start and stop, it's much harder to keep the momentum.

That's what happens in your brain when you're interrupted with an e-mail alert. You're working on a spreadsheet or document, and you get a little pop-up box or noise that you have a new message. You absolutely cannot resist the urge to check it. Now, be honest, out of every ten incoming e-mail messages you receive, how many are really important? One? Two? So you're forcing your brain to start/stop/start/stop constantly, effectively putting on the brakes and then giving more gas. All this effort requires a huge amount of mental energy.

▲ ENERGY BOOSTER | **Avoid Obsessive-Compulsive Technology Disorder**

Don't be a slave to the send/receive key, checking e-mail constantly throughout the day. Here's how to control yourself:

- Determine how often and what time you will check e-mail, such as once in the morning, once after lunch, and an hour before leaving work. Discipline yourself not to touch your e-mail outside of these specified periods. This will prevent you from getting sucked into the e-mail vortex for hours, drawn into an endless cycle of sending and receiving messages.
- If you have a hard time checking your e-mail only a few

times a day, bring an egg timer from home, shut down your e-mail program completely, set the timer for one hour, and do not check your e-mail until it goes off. If you can't do this, you need help. Discipline yourself to get work done.

- Be willing to turn off your BlackBerry to focus on a project.
- When you need some time to concentrate, turn on your voice mail, forward all calls, take your phone off the hook, hide your blinking light—do whatever you have to so that you're not disturbed by your phone. People are not going to die if they can't reach you for an hour. Those are expectations you are placing on yourself, rather than others placing them on you.
- Resist the temptation to peek at your e-mail one last time before taking a break, leaving the office for the day, or turning off the computer. That could result in thirty minutes of additional work.
- One of my clients, an executive assistant at Bank of America, set an out-of-office alert she kept on all the time that said, "I check e-mail around nine o'clock, noon, and three o'clock. If this is an emergency, please call me." I love that. She trained people how to treat her, and if they needed her right away, they learned to call.

▲ ▲ ▲
▼ ▼ ▼

▼ ENERGY BANDIT #7 | Instant messaging

I tried instant messaging at one point and immediately turned it off, since my productivity suffered terribly. I could be right in the middle of writing an article when *bing,* up popped a box with a message from a friend. Not that I didn't want to talk with her, but the message was much lower priority than what I was working on and took me off my important task. A recent study confirmed that instant

messaging and desktop alerts are terrible for concentration and productivity. You can lose all your energy just trying to concentrate on
a task while ignoring the dings and pop-up boxes. The findings from
this research suggest that instant-notification features be disabled to
avoid exacerbating the number of interruptions workers receive.[4]

▲ ENERGY BOOSTER | **Just say no to instant messaging**

Voice mail was invented to stave off the immediate interruption of
a ringing telephone. We have become pretty good at setting our
phone to send all calls to voice mail when we can't be disturbed. Enter instant messaging, which is ten times worse, because if you're online, you can be interrupted at any second. Here are some ways to
get a handle on it:

- Don't be afraid to turn on the "Do not disturb" or "Not
  available" feature on your IM when you have high energy
  and want to focus for thirty minutes on a task that requires
  your complete concentration.
- Compartmentalize the time that you're online. Be available
  online for only a fixed window of time every day, or while
  working on specific projects that require brainstorming with
  an off-site project partner.
- Be prepared to wind down a message session when it begins
  to develop a life of its own that drains your time.
- Seriously consider refusing to use this form of communication. Besides, instant messengers are just another possible entryway for computer security breaches.

▲　▲　▲

▼ ▼ ▼

| Using the wrong method of communication

How many times have you e-mailed back and forth with a coworker and thought, "If we just would have picked up the phone, we could have had this resolved by now"? Sometimes when a message requires dialogue or brainstorming or is complex, e-mail is not the best medium.

▲ ENERGY BOOSTER | Match the message to the medium

Of course, if you find yourself writing *War and Peace* in an e-mail, it might be better to pick up the phone. If the information you need to exchange is highly detailed, talking in person will ensure clarity. But if the information exchange necessitates brevity, then choose e-mail over telephone. Why? Because you have little control over how long a telephone conversation will last. You can drop hints about needing to end the conversation, but you never know if the person you're speaking to will pull a Chatty Cathy and tell a long, involved story about her grandson's latest sandbox escapades. And sometimes a colleague may launch into a discussion about a tangential project. Or maybe you'll be put on hold for five minutes because your client had another call coming in. Before you know it, you've spent twenty minutes on the phone, when you could have jotted your message down in three sentences in three minutes in an e-mail. Besides, if a miscommunication occurs, you'll have it in writing. If you order window envelopes instead of regular envelopes over the phone, and the printer prints the wrong ones, it's your word against theirs. But if it's in writing in an e-mail, you have proof and won't have to pay for the wrong envelopes.

▲ ▲ ▲

Nineteen

Purpose

Are you following your mission in life, or do you feel disconnected from what you want to do, believe in, and value? Are other people defining who you are? The more your time is organized around your values, the more energy you gain from your activities. Ian Percy, author of *Going Deep*, says, "When you are 'on purpose,' everything lines up and energy flows effortlessly and without restrictions." The key to purpose and energy is flow. Many people have pieces of their life that look great (e.g., a high-paying job, superior intellect, or a great family), but each great thing may not be enabling "flow." Anything short of flow and you spend lots of energy being restless and irritated. When what you believe in and what you do are in alignment, you'll experience higher satisfaction in everyday life. In this chapter, you'll explore your reality and your future. I'll show you how you can become congruent with your core values, spirituality, life balance, and time commitments in ways that give you boundless energy and happiness. You'll explore how to be who you really are, rather than trying to be like someone else or allowing others to define you.

▼ ▼ ▼

▼ ENERGY BANDIT #1 | Ignoring your dreams

When you were a little kid, what did you dream of becoming when you grew up? A writer? A photographer for *National Geographic*? A firefighter? Is that dream still lurking unfulfilled? Do you shrug off your deepest desires? Are you ignoring messages from the universe? Are you silencing your inner voice? Are you ignoring blissful recurring dreams?

For some reason, many of us have a deep-seated, perhaps even subconscious, belief that we don't *deserve* to achieve our dreams. Perhaps we think they're too pie-in-the-sky, too frivolous; we have to make a living, after all. We consciously or subconsciously thwart our efforts. It's almost as if we fear being happy.

Or maybe we're even a little lazy—it's much easier to plop down on the couch in front of the tube than to spend all your free time grinding toward a goal. There's no way around it: if you want to accomplish something in life, you have to exert some effort. Sure, all the atoms in the universe might be aligning themselves to flash very clear neon messages to you, but it's all for naught if you don't roll up your sleeves and put forth some effort to achieve your dreams.

▲ ENERGY BOOSTER | Figure out who *you* want to be and what *you* want to do

If you didn't have to worry about making money or about what anyone else would think, what would you do? Who do you want to be? What do you want to do? As Frank Sinatra sang, "Do be do be do." Spend a couple of hours in peaceful solitude to figure out what you want to do. Leave the spouse and kids at home. It's ideal if your outdoor place is fully furnished with a body of water—a lake, river, or stream. Stare at the water and listen to it. Sit by it. Meander along its banks. Visit this place several times over the next few weeks if you need to. You could also get away for an entire weekend by yourself. Rent a cabin in the woods or go camping. Don't take your laptop or BlackBerry, and leave your cell phone and watch in the glove compartment. While in this beautiful and peaceful setting, your job is to listen. Don't overanalyze. Don't think too hard. Simply let your thoughts gently wash over you like the soothing sound of the water. Start a journal. Write with a pen in your hand, not on the computer.

▲ ▲ ▲
▼ ▼ ▼

▼ ENERGY BANDIT #2 | The wrong career

Are you happy? Or are you just going through the motions to pay the bills? Do you find your work fulfilling? Of course there's a difference between everyday annoyances and unsettling, deep malcontent. People are people no matter where you go, and there will always be little problems no matter where you go. That's just life. I'm talking about a deep, undeniable sense of utter discontent and unhappiness. Life's too short to keep a job that makes your stomach hurt.

▲ ENERGY BOOSTER | Take a good, long look at your career choice

It takes some people years to finally get to their dream jobs. My mother wanted to open her own counseling center. She slowly took college classes in the evenings or during the day while we were at school. It was important to her to stay home until we got older, at which time she finally opened her practice. It's never too late—you can start anytime.

Do you ever experience a sense of panic about what you're *not* doing with your life through your work? This is often a midlife-crisis experience. But you don't have to wait until you're having a midlife crisis to figure out what you really should be doing with your life. As they say, do what you love, and the money will follow. To explore if you're in the right job:

- Make a list of your dreams. You may have only one; you may have several. Some may be really big. Some may be small. "I want to make jewelry and sell it online." "I want to be a meteorologist." "I want to start my own pension-consulting business."
- Make a list of your passions. What do you love? Singing? Playing guitar? Photography? Is there a dream job in there somewhere?
- Make a list of your core values. Is it important to you to have ample time to enjoy life? Is it important to you to be helping others through your work, no matter how many hours of the week it takes?
- Make a list of what you're naturally good at and love to do. Teaching people how to play tennis? Working with animals? Decluttering homes and offices? Cooking French cuisine? Is there a dream job in there somewhere?

▼ ENERGY BANDIT #3 | **Fear of following your dreams**

Perhaps you're afraid you won't make any money. Perhaps you're afraid to leave a high-paying job in search of a more fulfilling one. Perhaps you're afraid you'll fail. Whatever the reason, fear is a real energy drain. It will paralyze you, lock you up, and keep you in the status quo. If you are to find your purpose and experience the flow, you will have to muster the courage to fight it off.

▲ ENERGY BOOSTER | **Don't equate material success with achieving dreams**

Okay, so you have a BMW, a home with four bathrooms, your kids attend the best schools money can buy, and your wife looks like a supermodel. But you're unhappy, and you can't figure out why. Well, you know what they say: "Money can't buy happiness." And that's really it in a nutshell.

It's quite normal and understandable for people to want a lot of money. Having a lot of money, especially in a capitalistic society, is equivalent to having plenty. This is an instinctive, evolutionary drive. Of course you don't want to have to walk twenty miles with your Neanderthal club in hand to find a food source. But in a capitalistic society such as ours that's brimming with shiny *things*, this perfectly reasonable drive morphs into greed. And before you know it, we equate money and things with happiness.

But it's not money in and of itself that makes us happy. It's the *freedom* that money provides that opens a big, wide door to the land of happiness. In other words, if we're not living hand-to-mouth, we have the *time* to pursue what we truly love—whether that's writing a novel, volunteering full-time for a homeless shelter, or having time to watch the sun set every single evening.

How much did you spend on your most recently acquired boast-worthy possession? What if you were to take that same amount of money and donate it to a charity that feeds the hungry? Can you picture the poverty-stricken child whose face lights up when she receives a week's worth of hot meals? Which brings you more happiness, the possession or the child with a full stomach?

How do *you* like to make the world a better place? Helping people overcome illness? Working with the mentally handicapped? Teaching people how to exercise?

▲ ▲ ▲
▼ ▼ ▼

▼ ENERGY BANDIT #4 | Letting your obligations get in the way of your dreams

Sometimes the fear of a major overhaul, such as moving, makes us hesitate to achieve our dreams. And other times we have very valid, practical concerns, such as our children. But you are not your children. The day your children were born, your dreams did not cease to exist. Your children's dreams are theirs, not yours. You are here to encourage their dreams and help them attain them—but not to abandon yours in the meantime.

▲ ENERGY BOOSTER | Don't let the bills and the kids prevent you from pursuing your dreams

I've heard of people who moved to the geographic location of their dreams without jobs. And they found perfect jobs in their desired fields within just a few months. Of course, they saved plenty of money beforehand and worked temporary jobs once they arrived. The world isn't going to end if you have to wait tables at an upscale restaurant for sixty days. You'll have a lot of fun, and you'll be pleasantly surprised at how much money you can make doing that.

Yes, it may take a little bit longer to achieve your dreams than if you didn't have children, but being a parent is no reason to abandon your dreams. Don't you want to be a good role model for your children? Taking the initiative to achieve your dreams sends them a very healthy message about life and how to live it. Compartmentalize your time so that you have regular time to work toward your dreams; maybe that's after the kids are in bed or during soccer practice. You'll get there.

▲ ▲ ▲
▼ ▼ ▼

Spending time in ways that aren't important to you

During seminars, I often ask people about the most important things in their lives. They respond with the predictable: family, health, spirituality. Then I ask them, if I were to look at the way they spend their time, would I be able to tell what's important in their lives? Most people shake their heads. The majority of people spend far too much time working and not enough time with their loved ones. Then they arrive home and have no energy left to devote to their spouse or children. They take the day's problems out on the people they love—the entire reason they're working in the first place. You *say* your family is important to you. Can people tell you value them by the way you spend your time? You *say* your significant other is the most important thing in the world to you. How much time have you spent with him or her versus spending time working? You say your spirituality is important, but how much time do you spend praying, reading, meditating, attending services, volunteering, or whatever reflects your beliefs? Is it merely a facade? Say and do the same thing. Be congruent. Or just stop saying it and be yourself. To be in alignment with your values, what you say and what you do should be the same.

▲ ENERGY BOOSTER | **Adjust your life balance so your time reflects what matters to you most**

Put some metrics on your priorities. Companies measure their results, and you should measure yours. Spending time with my family is my greatest pleasure in life. Work is just my hobby. I want to be out of town only five nights per month. I want to eat dinner at home twenty-five days per month. I want to take six weeks of vacation each year. I work no more than forty-five hours per week, although I could easily work one hundred. Keeping track of my behavior each month makes me accountable; I know immediately whether my schedule is meshing with my priorities and my values. These figures are in front of me as a constant reminder of what I'm trying to accomplish with my life.

Assess how you're spending your time. What are you doing with it? Watching TV? Flipping through magazines? What would you rather be doing? What are your metrics going to be? What do you want your epitaph to say? "He had a well-mowed lawn"? "There wasn't one speck of dust in her house"? "His Porsche was really shiny"?

▲ ▲ ▲
▼ ▼ ▼

▼ ENERGY BANDIT #6 | Lack of a spiritual life

A study in the July 2006 issue of the *Journal of Mental Health Counseling* reported that spirituality (existential well-being) contributes greatly to life satisfaction.[1] Participants affirmed the importance of spirituality in life, stating that spirituality positively influenced their work behavior; helped them cope with stress at work; contributed positively to life satisfaction; and gave them a sense of hope, strength, and peace.

▲ ENERGY BOOSTER | Cultivate awareness of and faith in a greater power

People refer to their spiritual or higher power in different terms: God, spirit, Prana, Allah, the Lord, or the universe. I am a Christian and thank Jesus Christ for the blessings in my life. When things go well, I know that God is opening doors for me. However, you don't have to subscribe to a particular faith to be a spiritual person or to benefit from a daily dose of energy from your spiritual practice of choice.

Have you noticed that when things are going the way they should, they flow naturally along the path of least resistance? One way to confirm this is by looking back at your life. Are there things in your life that just seemed to magically "click" into place? Like the fact that my husband, John, and I met at a volleyball party hosted by two separate friends, who were roommates, at a house neither of us had ever been to. We both knew immediately we had met the right one. It was as if I had known him all my life.

Look back at the little puzzle pieces of the good things in your life to see how they fit together. If you have very few such little puzzle pieces that clicked into place seemingly by magic, perhaps you're ignoring the universe's messages and making poor choices. Don't go against the flow. Go *with* the flow. The flow is that little voice deep inside you. Listen to it in these ways, and see if the external world begins to follow suit:

- Open your eyes to synchronicity. The term *synchronicity* was coined by Swiss psychologist Carl Jung; he defined it as the product of all human minds working synergistically within the collective unconscious. This is in alignment with the scientific notion that thought waves can influence outcomes. Synchronicity can be interpreted as receiving little messages from the universe. For example, you finally say out loud, "I want to be a writer." Then the very next day you meet the head of a publishing company at a business luncheon. The trick is to be *aware* of such situations, and to act on them accordingly. But don't make the mistake of interpreting every single event as synchronicity, or you'll end up confusing yourself. You want to open your eyes to those messages that are loud and clear instead of shrugging them off with cynicism.

- Listen to repeated messages. Has the fourteenth person this week told you that you would be a great comedian—and it's something you've always wanted to do, but you just keep telling yourself that it's too hard to make it in show biz? If you keep receiving the same message over and over, listen to and then act on it. You may not become Eddie Murphy overnight, but you very well may get a regular gig at your local comedy club. And that can lead to bigger gigs, if that's where you want your life to go. Everyone has to start somewhere.

- Pray. Put it out there. Just ask for it. You don't have to believe in God to pray. It may take a few months or a few years to come back to you, but it will. There's a saying that goes something like "The universe rearranges itself to accommodate your view of reality."

▲ ▲ ▲
▼ ▼ ▼

▼ ENERGY BANDIT #7 | **Trying to be what others want you to be**

Maybe you chose to be an attorney because that's what your parents wanted you to be; your father is an attorney, and your grandfather was an attorney who founded the family-based practice. But deep inside you always wanted to be a schoolteacher. You knew your family expected you to continue the tradition and become a partner in the firm. Besides, you know that attorneys make a relatively good salary and it's generally a reputable career. But you really wanted to be a teacher: you love kids and have this almost magical way of helping them learn and understand things. All your nieces and nephews flock to you during family holiday get-togethers because they know they can talk you into doing something fun.

▲ ENERGY BOOSTER | **Avoid people who shatter your dreams**

I've seen a bumper sticker that says "Those who abandon their dreams will discourage yours." Avoid them like the plague. And don't believe a word they say. Yes, you *can* do it.

Did you see the movie about Johnny Cash called *Walk the Line?* Johnny Cash's father incessantly belittled Johnny's childhood dream of becoming a singer someday, despite his obvious talent. In the movie, Johnny has made it big and invites his parents to his new home for Thanksgiving. His father quickly glances around the house and says that Jack Benny's house is better. Johnny doesn't miss a beat. He replies, "Have you ever been in Jack Benny's house?" Johnny Cash is the perfect example of how to never, ever listen to people who put down your dreams, and to believe in yourself and work hard to attain them instead. This persistence helped him become a legend in his own lifetime.

Of course, this is a little easier said than done. Dream dashing by our parents, teachers, and "friends" can have a harmful effect upon us. Our bodies can internalize these hurtful messages. Here's what to do to achieve your dreams:

- If your "friends," coworkers, or family members chronically pooh-pooh or laugh off your dreams, politely but firmly explain to them that this is very important to you, and that you would appreciate it if they would support you rather than discourage you.
- Surround yourself with people who encourage your dreams. And reciprocate by supporting their dreams.
- Are you a budding entrepreneur who could benefit from a strong support network of like-minded professionals? Join or start a Mastermind group. The Mastermind concept was developed by Napoleon Hill in the early 1900s in his book *Think and Grow Rich*. Members of a Mastermind group further one another's success by reporting success achieved

since the last meeting, collectively brainstorming solutions to any problems a member may be experiencing, and holding each member accountable for achieving his or her goals. It doesn't matter if you're starting your dream business or trying to attain spiritual transcendence. Mastermind groups are simply for like-minded individuals with similar goals, who will offer practical advice and even *push* one another to achieve their stated goals.

▲ ▲ ▲
▼ ▼ ▼

▼ ENERGY BANDIT #8 | Being all talk and no action

I know a woman who finally has her dream job; it took her fourteen years to get there. After working in marketing for years to put bread on the table, she's now a freelance writer. But when her husband would introduce her to others, he'd say that she was a consultant. During the drive home after one such event, she finally said to her husband, "Are you ashamed of what I do for a living?" Her husband, perplexed, replied, "No, why?" She said, "Because you keep introducing me as a consultant. I'm not a consultant. I'm a *Freelance Writer*." He got the message loud and clear—including capitalization of the words *Freelance* and *Writer*, given the emphasis in her voice— that it was very important to her to be recognized, finally, as what she had always wanted to be.

▲ ENERGY BOOSTER | Claim your dream

Grab a piece of paper and a pen. Without overanalyzing, act straight from your gut and finish this sentence: I am a _____. Now say it aloud to yourself. Does it have a nice ring? Does it make you smile? Does it make you feel happy? Does it make you giggle? Does it make you want to raise your arms skyward in exaltation and exclaim for the entire world to hear, over and over again, "I am a _____."

Now you'll have to make those dreams a reality. You've always dreamed of being a novelist? You're going to have to insert regular writing time into your schedule. You may even want to attend a writer's retreat, take a writer's class, or join a local writing group. You'll have to educate yourself about how to properly prepare and solicit your manuscript. And if you get rejected, you'll have to pull up your boot straps and try it again. And again. And again.

Working toward your dreams could involve all matter of practical tasks: saving money, getting an education, moving, and working a temporary second job. Without effort, dreams are only hollow wishes. There's a quaint saying from the South: "Wishin' don't paint the porch."

▲ ▲ ▲

Twenty

Workplace

Periphery quiz item #20:
Stop the meeting. I want to get off!

The workplace is full of energy drains, even for people who work at home. You open Outlook and get sucked into the e-mail vortex. You open your Internet browser and spend an hour surfing, and then realize you have a headache. A coworker drops by to chat, and you can literally feel your energy drain as he drones on and on. You attend a meeting where minutes are taken but much time is wasted. Lo and behold, hours have passed, and you've expended precious energy without much return. In this chapter, you'll look at how much you allow external interruptions to dictate your schedule. You'll figure out how to keep your typical distractions at bay and prevent disruptions and disturbances. I'll help you eliminate your excuses, build barriers, create preventive assertions, and challenge your thinking. We'll try to create situations that are suited to concentrated, focused work without interruptions.

▼ ▼ ▼

▼ ENERGY BANDIT #1 | **Understaffing and overcommitment**

When my husband, John, and I had our first child in 2000, he left his job as a letter carrier at the United States Postal Service and came to work in our business. Admittedly, this was a difficult transition for him. As a letter carrier, your work is self-evident. In the morning, you have a big pile of mail. At the end of the day, it's gone. And if you try to take your work home with you, they will come and find you. It's finished. Complete. It has a beginning and an end. He worked hard, but if he had too much mail, it waited for the next day. Now, as the COO of our company, it's tougher for him to "finish." He now has a lot more ideas about what to do to grow our company than time to do it. How about you? Do you have more things to do than time to do them? Do your tasks seem to pile up faster each day? Have you ever finished? Most people haven't. As a result, they often lie awake at night with all those to-dos running around in their heads.

Not only do you have a lot on your plate, but you often inherit the work of someone who leaves, is downsized, or goes on parental leave or short-term disability. Many organizations don't replace those jobs but simply split up the tasks of people who leave and divvy them up among a few others. Or simply give the job to one person, requiring that poor sap to do the work of all three. It's no wonder people don't have the energy to drag themselves out of bed and head to the office each day. If you have too much to do and too little time to do it, your job is interfering with your personal life, you work on your own time, or the sheer volume of work interferes with how well you do it, you are on track for burnout.

▲ ENERGY BOOSTER | **Speak up when you have too much on your plate**

Try the following verbal techniques to call attention to overwork:

- Negotiate to extend the deadline. Say something like, "Do you need that today, or would Monday be okay?"

- Simplify and try to reduce the scope of the task. "At what level of detail does this need to be done?"
- Communicate by being honest about what's on your plate. "Here's a list of the things I'm working on in priority order. Where would you say this falls?"
- Reduce quality. Can the task be done at 85 percent rather than 100 percent perfect? "What level of perfection is required here?"
- Delegate. Can you form a committee? Can you hire a contractor? "Can I get help on this, or do I need to do it myself?"
- Streamline by doing it more efficiently or changing a process. "Can we skinny this down a bit?"
- Get creative. How else could you meet the request? Suggest an alternative way to get the result, other than what the boss outlined or the way you're doing it now. "It might be more efficient if I had access to your calendar, rather than sending you an e-mail or calling you."
- Partial delivery. Can you do a piece now and pieces later? Set milestones for delivery. "I can get this first part done today and get the rest to you by Friday."
- Redirect by asking the requester to send it to someone else if it doesn't belong on your plate. "That request actually goes through IT; I'll make sure they know about this problem."

▼ ENERGY BANDIT #2 | **Wanting to feel needed**

Everyone wants you in his or her meeting. You are the power broker. Your in-box is full of meeting requests, all of which you accept. Your calendar is so full of people wanting a piece of you that you have no time left to work. Sound familiar?

▲ ENERGY BOOSTER | Be unavailable

That's right. When someone says, "Do you have a minute?" it's okay to say, "Not right now." You don't have to be rude or impolite, but you do have to be honest. Over the years, you have trained people how to treat you, and you're giving a lesson right this very second. If your behavior shouts, "I'm available at all times, so bother me," you will never have a moment's peace; everything and everyone will be vying for your attention. How do you keep those distractions, pop-in visitors, and interruptions at bay? By managing your availability, you will gain the space of time and mind to complete your most important tasks.

You can say, "I do want to talk with you about this, and I'm buried in another deadline right now. Can I call you at ten o'clock tomorrow?" Or you can push back by saying (without sarcasm), "I have just one minute. Are you sure that's all you'll need?" Do not smile. When the person says, "Oh, uh, well, actually, maybe ten minutes," then you can say, "Oh, in that case I'll need to ask you to set up some time to chat. I'm right in the middle of a train of thought and want to give my full attention to what you're discussing." Unless it's your job to be interrupted (receptionist, customer-service phone operator, administrative assistant, and so forth), then it's acceptable not to respond to everyone's beck and call. Come up with some sort of signal with your team that indicates to everyone else that now is not a good time. It can be a flag, a sign, a banner, or any other physical cue that tells coworkers you're busily concentrating on a task. Have an understanding that if there's an emergency, coworkers can still feel free to interrupt, but if they were simply coming by for a little social interaction or a question that isn't pressing, the signal tells them to please come back later. Here are some other methods to manage your availability:

- For meetings, unless you see a clear agenda with the objectives and outcome and the specific reason you are being invited to it, decline the request (unless it's your boss). Don't let people get away with inviting you just in case. Make sure the meeting purpose is a good return on your time investment. Get out of as many meetings as possible.

- If your presence is required for only a small portion of the meeting, call the meeting leader. Ask for your report to be first on the agenda. After speaking and answering questions, leave.

- Push the value of the meeting down to the lowest common denominator and send your assistant, if at all possible, in your stead. First, think about the length of the particular meeting you've been invited to. Second, think about the cost of that meeting, given your salary level. Third, think about the opportunity cost, in terms of what you could do instead of attending the meeting. Fourth, think about whether your assistant is capable and knowledgeable enough to sit in on the meeting. Fifth, contemplate whether you've given him or her enough authority to be able to take an agenda item off the table. It's frustrating for meeting attendees to hear from your delegate, "I'll have to check with so-and-so and get back to you." They would much rather hear, "I can absolutely ensure that will happen and can have the results to you by Thursday."

- I once taught a seminar where someone told me he is invited to meetings because people don't want to hurt his feelings by not including him. He just sits there with no input and can't figure out why his presence was requested. There should be open communication about attendance; when necessary, say that you don't feel you need to be there and ask if your attendance is required.

▲ ▲ ▲

▼ ▼ ▼

▼ ENERGY BANDIT #3 | Being unprepared for meetings

My favorite Chance card in Monopoly is "Get out of Jail Free." Wouldn't it be nice if you could have a "Get out of a Meeting Free" card? That would be worth a mint.

Meetings and social events at work are a central fact of organizational life. As a vehicle for communication, they can be extremely valuable mechanisms for disseminating vision, crafting strategic plans, and developing responses to challenges and opportunities. They can also be helpful for gathering ideas, brainstorming, and generating higher levels of employee involvement. But too many meetings, where time is wasted and no decisions are made, are a source of energy drain.

▲ ENERGY BOOSTER | Prepare to have a great meeting

The productivity of any meeting actually starts before the meeting begins. These planning elements determine whether or not the meeting will be a success:

- Require an agenda twenty-four hours in advance, with the responsible person and the time listed next to each item, in order of priority. A statement of the purpose for the meeting should be included.
- If it's a conference call with participants in different time zones, put people in later time zones at the beginning of the agenda.
- Ensure that all invitees really need to be there.
- Send a delegate in your place if the person is capable of making decisions and can sign off on or take responsibility for completing a task. Let the leader know you're sending someone.

- Distribute materials twenty-four hours in advance. State what people are expected to bring or report on.
- Meetings should end fifteen minutes before the top of the hour, to allow people to get to the next meeting without being late.
- Match the importance and complexity of the issue to the length of the meeting.
- Meet for issues involving discussion only, not FYI items.
- Come prepared and read advance materials.

▲ ▲ ▲
▼ ▼ ▼

▼ ENERGY BANDIT #4 | Chaos during meetings

The meeting drags on too long. There are side conversations. People are tapping e-mails on their BlackBerries while someone is talking. The discourtesies abound. You spend ninety minutes in what should have been a forty-five-minute meeting and leave with your energy flagging and frustrated.

▲ ENERGY BOOSTER | Create a meeting code of conduct

The next time you attend a staff or committee meeting, request the opportunity to lead an exercise aimed at making meetings more productive and less draining. Tell the group you would like to discuss some guidelines and protocols about meetings. Standing in front of a flip chart, ask the group, "If you were king or queen of the world, what rules would you make about meetings, to make them as productive as possible? What makes you crazy about our meetings? How do we waste time?" and list the statements people make. Type these up, title it "Code of Conduct," put it on a piece of 8½ × 11-inch paper, and take it to a print shop to be blown up into a poster-sized piece of paper. Frame it and hang it in the meeting rooms to remind people about proper behavior in a meeting. Following are some sample guidelines:

- If the leader or key decision maker no-shows, attendees may leave after ten minutes.
- Use a timekeeper (appointed by the leader) to keep the meeting on target and follow the agenda.
- Appoint a scribe for the meeting. When something comes up that's not on the agenda, the scribe records it on the flip chart. If there is time at the end of the meeting, those items can be addressed. If time runs out, they roll over to the next meeting agenda.
- Action items are recorded as "who/what/when" on a flip chart. The scribe types these up after the meeting and distributes them within forty-eight hours.
- Meetings will start and stop on time, unless all in attendance agree to extend the time.
- Try to finish early if possible; don't stretch the meeting.
- Attendees may get up and leave at the stated end time.
- Eliminate any discussion that involves only two people.
- Don't stop meetings to bring latecomers up-to-date.

▲ ▲ ▲
▼ ▼ ▼

▼ ENERGY BANDIT #5 | Coworkers constantly interrupt your flow

You're right in the middle of a great train of thought on a creative-writing project, and a peer pops his head into your office and, without waiting to be acknowledged, starts talking. You glance up, about to ask if he can come back, when you realize you have lost your idea anyway.

▲ ENERGY BOOSTER | Schedule your interruptions

Perhaps one of the reasons you're being interrupted so frequently is you're never around and available. This is especially true of people who travel for a living or spend most of the day wrapped up in meetings. It's understandable that you'll be pounced upon by your assistant when you suddenly emerge, because she's been waiting to ask you questions for two days. Here are some ways you can actually plan for and around interruptions:

- Schedule regular check-in times. If you have an assistant, you'll want to set up a regular time (or several times) each day or week to touch base. Have your assistant save up all the questions he or she has and ask them all at once during your regularly scheduled meeting. This process keeps your assistant from interrupting you ten times a day to ask you one thing and instead uses one meeting to ask you ten things. Similarly, if your boss is the one you aren't able to pin down, suggest this process for yourself.

- Block out interruptible times. One human resources director I worked with figured out that she was interrupted every eleven minutes. Although talking with employees was important, she had to work late just to get her work done because she couldn't get the space of mind to finish a task through completion. I suggested she block out several time periods each day and ask people to "sign up" instead. She scheduled an "Interruption" block in her Outlook calendar from 9:00 to 11:00 and 1:00 to 3:00 each day, printed her calendar sheets, and taped them to the counter of the reception area. Her assistant fielded interruptions, telling employees she now scheduled discussions by appointment, and people willingly checked the blocks of time and signed up for a thirty-minute meeting. If it was an absolute emergency (the HR director had already briefed her assistant on what issues were deemed an emergency), the appointment was waived. Perhaps you won't block out four hours a day as she did, but you can use the concept to communicate to peers, internal customers, and subordinates the times you're willing to be interrupted. Think of it as a limited "open door" policy: only open at certain times. You might think it won't work, but would you expect your hairstylist to allow you to drop by when she's not working? Would you then get upset that she didn't respond to your beck and call? Believe me, people will get used to it.

- Set aside downtime. One architecture firm I worked with established a firm no-interruption time during the hours of 9:00 to 10:30 every morning. How would you like to have ninety minutes of complete concentration every day, when meetings aren't allowed, instant messaging is disabled, phones are forwarded to voice mail, no interruptions are allowed, and the e-mail servers are turned off? Drastic? But *wildly* popular for the people who could actually focus on completing an important task without being distracted. You probably won't be able to swing this policy company-wide, but you could try to work it out with those whom you work with most. You are probably interrupted by a core group of people throughout the day, so work with your team to establish this downtime, dedicated to real work.

- Attach a big STOP sign to your cubicle entry and wear your headset (possibly without any music—people will think you're listening to something). When crunch time comes, all you have to do is turtle up and leave a note on your door explaining the situation. Or tape a big X with masking tape across the entry with a sign saying, IF YOU INTERRUPT ME, THERE HAD BETTER BE BLOOD INVOLVED.

▲ ▲ ▲

▼ ▼ ▼

| Being unwilling to challenge things that waste your time

Many company policies don't make any sense but still waste inordinate amounts of time and energy. It reminds me of the story of the little girl who was watching her mother prepare their holiday ham. She unwrapped and cleaned it, sliced the ends off, and put it in the pan. She put cloves, pineapple, and cherries on it and put it in the oven. The little girl asked, "Mommy, why did you cut the ends off the ham?" The mother replied, "Because my mother always did. Let's call her and find out." So they called Grandma and asked the same question. "Hmmm, that's a good one. You'll have to call Momma and ask." So the mother put in a call to the elderly great-grandmother of the little girl. "Nanna, why did you cut the ends off the ham?" "Why, dear," replied the old woman, "my pan wasn't big enough to hold it." Do you ever hear "That's just the way we've always done it" at your company, even if it defies all logic?

▲ ENERGY BOOSTER | Challenge the status quo

Some of the company rules you must abide by don't make any sense. For years, I've heard employees in my productivity seminars complain about their information technology (IT) departments. I believe some of these complaints have valid justifications, and in those cases I stick up for IT. For example, "IT won't let me load personal software on my machine or visit the sites I want to see" has a justified reason, since doing so would create a staffing nightmare as workers seek help on nonsupported applications. It could also create security concerns and open the door to system viruses. Restricting certain Internet sites makes sense, as I just can't think of a good reason why employees would need to watch X-rated videos at work.

However, not having a desktop printer is a major pain, an energy drain, and a productivity sucker. Having to walk down the hall to the printer is the most ridiculous thing I've heard of in a while. Holy cow, I print continually. Even those with handheld devices still have piles of paper all over their desks. It's crazy to think about how much people make per hour times the number of employees in an organization, all walking down the hall to the shared printer, where of course they're likely to stumble into Chatty Suzy, who wants to tell you about the latest flowers blooming in her garden. You get to the printer—darn it, it didn't print out; someone accidentally took my stuff with theirs; it's not what I thought I printed; the margins are cut off; and so forth—BACK to the office to print again. I don't care about how hard it is to service all those printers. Get a contractor to handle it. Printers are cheap. The cost of not having a printer on the desktop of every employee is a huge productivity and profitability drain. If they won't buy one for you, bring your own. Keep yelling. Keep complaining. I know of several employees who made enough of a fuss that the policy was actually changed just for them.

▼ ENERGY BANDIT #7 | **Not having the tools you need to get the job done efficiently**

Although you don't want to be checking your BlackBerry constantly while you're at home with your family, it does come in handy while you're traveling. I love being able to get my e-mail while I'm in a taxi on the way to the hotel and clear out my in-box. When I return to my office after the trip, I don't have hundreds of e-mails piled up. But perhaps your job description doesn't fit some predefined requirement on who gets a handheld and who doesn't.

▲ ENERGY BOOSTER | Argue for the tools and equipment you need

Due to the nature of your job, you might be far more productive if you had instant access to your company's e-mail, calendar, and contacts when you're on the road. You will need to build a business case about how a handheld will improve your productivity level and present it to your boss. Upon your return, you would have more energy to do other work rather than wade through your e-mail. Additionally, if your personality and job situation are more suited to electronic means, you'd waste less time and energy searching for things than in a paper system. You might be forced to print your Outlook calendar, schlep it home, write on it manually, and carry it back to work to update it again, just to keep things organized. If you absolutely can't get your boss to buy you a handheld, suck it up and buy it yourself.

Many organizations are out of touch with the business reality of what their workers are dealing with. For example, I've actually seen a policy where employees were not allowed to load personal information in Outlook. Ridiculous. People don't simply turn off their private lives when they walk through their office door, and they don't stop thinking about work at home, either. Keep stamping your feet and speaking up loudly until you're heard. The expression "The squeaky wheel gets the grease" is very true here. If you're sick of hiking down the hall to the shared printer to get your printouts, request your own local printer. If they say no, go to your boss, then go to his boss, then go to the IT manager—go to anyone who will listen. When you provide a valid business justification and show how much money they are wasting by making you walk to your printouts, you'll be far more likely to get your way.

▲   ▲   ▲

▼ ▼ ▼

| **Repetitiveness and redundancy**

Once you've performed a task several times, you have the luxury of trying to figure out how to do it more efficiently with less energy exerted.

▲ ENERGY BOOSTER | **Become more efficient and get things done more quickly**

Some tasks that are done over and over again can be done more efficiently. Here are some questions to ask yourself:

- Can you create a checklist to handle repetitive tasks quickly? Before I leave for a speaking engagement, I have to know that certain things are in place: books are shipped, travel arrangements are made, workbook copies have been produced, an LCD projector will be available, and so forth. So we automated the process of providing this information to me. At the time of the booking, each staff person includes a checklist in the central client hard-copy file and marks things off as they are accomplished and put in the file. I simply have to pull the file, scan the checklists, and see what's been done and any exceptions. It ensures that each person completes all the necessary tasks prior to an engagement, and I don't have to ask whether things have been completed.
- Can you lower your standards? Does it have to be done perfectly? I worked with the president of a car manufacturing company who called someone in IT to get a figure to put into his presentation. The president was thinking the guy would spend fifteen minutes on it and be able to quickly ballpark a number to drop into his speech. Turns out the employee

spent ten hours coming up with an exact number to seven digits, when the president was looking for only a high-level guess—5 million or 50 million? Both of them were at fault. The president should have said, "I'm looking for this type of number, and I'm thinking it will just take you fifteen minutes or so to ballpark it plus or minus a few million dollars. Does that sound reasonable?" Then the employee could have told him how much time it would actually take to come up with that figure and the president could have decided if it was worth it for that particular speech.

- Can you use a shortcut? How about a standard response template? I found myself responding to the same types of e-mails and providing the same information over and over again, such as replying to media requests for quotes, thanking people for kind feedback to a presentation, sending invoices, and so forth. I used to keep standard templates in Microsoft Word and cut and paste them into Outlook. But I have saved SO much time by setting up the standard templates as "Signatures" in Microsoft Outlook and titling them by the type of response or letter. I simply create or reply to the e-mail, hit insert, then signature, then pick the name of the signature, customize a couple of things, and hit send. Simple! What a great shortcut.

▲ ▲ ▲

Twenty-one

Clutter

Periphery quiz item #21:
Can I get rid of my relatives?

Look around you, at work and at home. Do you feel overjoyed or annoyed? Your environment affects your moods, attitudes, emotions, and energy levels. What things sap your energy? When you get dressed in the morning, can you quickly find something to wear? Or do you have a bunch of clothes that don't fit you, so you walk out thinking you're "fat"? How does your stuff affect you? In this chapter, you'll look at your space, possessions, and memories to find the energy bandits in your surroundings. I'll help you figure out ways to reduce, eliminate, or change your environment, so it lifts you up rather than brings you down.

▼ ▼ ▼

▼ ENERGY BANDIT #1 | Cluttered surroundings

Feng shui, pronounced "fung schway," is the Chinese art of placement—but it goes far beyond simple interior decorating. *Feng* means "wind" and *shui* means "water." Feng shui is the arrangement of space to attain harmony with the natural environment; it is a geoscience concerned with how the surrounding environment affects human life. The overarching goal of feng shui is to orient property, dwellings, and even possessions in optimum alignment with energy. And guess what one of the number-one concepts of feng shui is? "Avoid clutter."[1]

Yes, clearing away clutter requires diligent effort and can be time-consuming. But the *real* reason people dread clearing clutter is due to emotional attachment—the love letters you kept from failed relationships, the old receipts from trips, brochures from concerts—and no idea how to organize what you keep. Clearing clutter isn't just about achieving tidiness; it's actually an emotional process that's akin to therapy. Thus, it requires a healthy dose of stamina. But once you clear your clutter and keep it away, you'll experience clarity, a sense of well-being, and remarkably high energy levels.[2]

▲ ENERGY BOOSTER | **Prioritize your decluttering mission in feng shui order**

When you're clearing the clutter, focus first on the areas of the home that are most important to your health and vitality:

- Focus on your bedroom first. We are most strongly influenced by people, items, and events that are closest to us, so the bedroom is the most important room in the home. Clear out the space under your bed. Do not store items under your bed.
- Then clean out your closet and drawers. Chuck anything you haven't worn in two years; put it in your charity box or bag. Ditto for anything that's too tight. The washing and drying process makes clothes shrink over time. Besides, clothes that are too tight sap your energy by restricting circulation and making you feel fat. Your clothes can also become tight in different places after you've begun exercising every day; that's because you're replacing squishy fat with toned muscle. It's okay to keep some silly things from past decades, as they'll be handy at costume parties or fabulously retro in just a few years.

- Organize what you keep by seasons so that you can find your clothing easily. For example, hang all short-sleeved shirts together, and hang all long-sleeved shirts together. You can even move items when seasons change so you can locate them more quickly.

- Remove any visual and energy clutter that doesn't belong in the bedroom. This includes children's toys or items, exercise equipment, paperwork, the television, and the computer.[3] An adult bedroom is for sleeping and intimate relationships, and everything in the bedroom should be on that wavelength. Decorate the nightstand with romantic candles, not bills to pay.

- Next, declutter the kitchen. The kitchen represents your state of health. It is especially associated with your liver, which is the organ primarily responsible for detoxifying the body. Start with the fridge. Get rid of those leftovers that are growing eyeballs and the fossilized jelly. Then remove everything from the fridge and wipe it down with warm, soapy water. Ditto for the freezer. Are you really going to eat that chunk of freezer-burned anniversary cake that's been in there for five years? Next, deep-clean the stove. Don't use toxic cleansers with harsh chemicals. Opt instead for citrus-based degreasers, such as Citra-Solv. Check your local health-food store's natural cleaning products or visit the Seventh Generation Web site at www.seventhgeneration.com.

- Then clean out all cabinets and drawers. If you never use it, donate it to charity. That goes for food items too; they can be donated to the local soup kitchen, food bank, or a local church. Organize what you do keep. Last, clean all counter surfaces and light fixtures.[4]

- Now it's time to clear the main entrance. In feng shui, your main entrance is where your home receives its primary energy. When you enter any dwelling, your energy is looking for grounding and focus; therefore, having a clutter-free entryway provides visual relief. Move any unnecessary items out of the entryway, such as recycling bins or stacks of mail. Recycling bins can be tucked under the kitchen sink, in the kitchen pantry, or, better yet, in the garage. Keep only in-season items in the coat closet; place the rest in storage. Infuse your entryway with a sense of beauty; try adding a houseplant.[5]

▲ ▲ ▲
▼ ▼ ▼

▼ ENERGY BANDIT #2 | A nonstop flow of new stuff

Perhaps you just can't resist a good bargain. Maybe you go to garage sales for fun. Whatever the reason, there's a constant stream of new possessions that manages to find a way into your home. Americans have so much stuff, we have to rent storage space. We park our cars outside and fill our garages with junk. Just what every American needs—more *stuff*. When you start saying no to more stuff, you'll experience an undeniable feeling of freedom—not to mention being able to save more of your money for the really important intangible "things" in life, such as your child's college education or your retirement. Don't feel obligated to keep something you don't like just because it was a gift. Selling items on eBay is a great way to unload unwanted or duplicate gifts.

▲ ENERGY BOOSTER | Thin out the constant incoming stream

If you don't develop a regular habit of thinning this stuff as it comes through the door, it will pile up and zap your energy in no time. Keep your junk to a minimum by following these tips:

- As soon as you bring in the mail, sort it. Keep what you need, and recycle what you don't need. Right then and there.

Don't leave the mail in a sloppy pile on the kitchen counter, or you'll always be staring at a to-do item, which will increase your feelings of being overwhelmed and fatigued. File bills in a chronological stack in your desk. Pay your bills one night a week. It will sap your energy if you save the stack for later. Taking thirty seconds to sort your mail now is much, much easier than wading through it for an entire hour one week later.

- As soon as you arrive home with unwanted gifts from your holiday gatherings, return or exchange what you can, give them to charity, or sell them on eBay.

- Don't feel obligated to take home a carload of junk when you visit your parents over the holidays. For some reason, some parents, no matter what age their grown children are, feel the need to equip them with carloads of more *stuff* when they come to visit. If your parents fall into this category, resolve to yourself today to just say no the next time you visit them. But if there's space in the car and it's a truly valuable item, you could take it home and sell it on eBay. Shhh. I won't tell.

- Do you find that you can't resist something that's on sale even though you don't need it? Approach yard sales and clearance sales with extreme caution. Don't buy it if you don't like it, no matter how great a deal it is.

- Draw a distinct line between wants and needs. Eschew impulsive buying at the checkout counter. The next time you want to buy something, question whether it is a want or a need and sleep on major purchases.

▲ ▲ ▲

▼ ▼ ▼

▼ ENERGY BANDIT #3 | **Not having the right organizational tools and equipment**

You could be buried in clutter simply because you don't know where to put things.

▲ ENERGY BOOSTER | **Create space with the right layout and equipment**

Ample space gives us peace of mind; clutter makes us feel irritable and overwhelmed. Take back control with these clutter busters:

- Use vertical space instead of horizontal space. Look up. People all too often forget to use vertical space. This is particularly true in the garage. Install shelving. Organize all those piles of books and CDs lying on the floor and put them on shelves.
- Purchase what you need to organize your belongings efficiently: photo albums, a shredder, file cabinets, file folders, a desk, bookshelves, and storage containers. Map out an area, determining where you need a storage solution. Visit Web sites such as www.elfa.com and organizing stores such as The Container Store before you go shopping.
- Measure your space and determine what will fit before you go shopping. Put things away. Your treasures belong in cabinets, drawers, and closets—not on the floor, on counters, or on tabletops. Do you have a pile of newspapers on the living room floor? Recycle them. Do you keep your mail piled on the kitchen counter? Toss all the junk mail, put the bills out of sight in your desk, and file long-term documents in your filing cabinet. Any items on furniture surfaces in the bed-

room should be decorative or highly functional in nature, such as an alarm clock or a lamp. Put the pile of dirty laundry on the floor in the dirty-clothes hamper, and put the clean laundry away. The kitchen counter is not the place to create a to-do pile; keep bills and larger items that you need to mail in a tickler file in your desk. Keeping piles on the kitchen counter also makes you less likely to wipe down the counter, resulting in an area that is both untidy and dirty.

▲ ▲ ▲
▼ ▼ ▼

▼ ENERGY BANDIT #4 | Owning too many possessions

All too often in the United States, people equate material possessions with wealth, happiness, and, worse yet, self-worth. This reminds me of a T-shirt I've seen. It has a 1950s woman on it, and she's saying, "I'd like more *things*, please." We're subconsciously afraid that people will judge us not only by the house we live in and the car we drive but by the types of belongings we acquire. Add to this the fact that *things* are relatively inexpensive in the United States, and before you know it, your house is bursting at the seams with possessions.

Not only does the clutter of material possessions drain your energy, but spending too much of your money on possessions will also drain your pocketbook. And a drained pocketbook will deplete your energy even more.

▲ ENERGY BOOSTER | Don't be too materialistic; decide to live more simply

• Take a long, hard look at your decorative items. Do you have an entire wall filled with photos of family members? Be selective about wall hangings. Ample wall space also exudes peace of mind. You just can't quit acquiring antique chairs from flea markets, most of which go completely unused? Keep your most prized models, and then sell the rest in a special antique-oriented yard sale. Or you could place an ad in the newspaper, which will attract a lot of serious buyers.

- Keep your collectibles in check. Do you really need another piece of memorabilia from the seventies rock band Kiss? Is your guest room starting to look like the Rock and Roll Hall of Fame? If you have a small roadside museum in a small tourist town that people pay admission to see, that's one thing, but unnecessary clutter is entirely different. Keep your favorite paraphernalia, and get rid of the rest.

- Before the holidays, guide your children in donating to charity toys they no longer play with; this also teaches them the joy of giving. Have younger children try on clothes each season to see what they've outgrown; give the clothes to younger friends or family members, or donate them. Continue this cycle with teenagers; although they may not outgrow clothing as quickly, they stop using and wearing certain items.

▲ ▲ ▲
▼ ▼ ▼

▼ ENERGY BANDIT #5 | **Being afraid to get rid of things**

Perhaps your parents said, "Don't throw anything away! Everything has value." And you're still holding on to those beliefs. While necessary during the Great Depression, that type of thinking today will create a society of pack rats who can't throw anything away but desperately need to. The underlying drive behind this behavior is an excessive concern that a given object shouldn't be discarded, as it might be needed later. This behavior can also include excessive acquisition, such as compulsive shopping, extreme collecting, or hoarding free items, such as catalogs or junk mail. Acquisition behavior indicates extreme indecisiveness about what to keep; the indecisiveness is so extreme that the hoarder completely avoids the decision-making process and ends up keeping everything. Then the hoarder experiences difficulty figuring out how to organize all the kept items.[6]

Sometimes hoarding behavior becomes severe. Not only can it extend to the office and one's vehicle, but fire marshals have even declared such residences a fire hazard. In one extreme case, a hoarder rented a second apartment to live in because his own had grown too full of belongings. This behavior is more common in men than in women. If your behavior is severe—such as having to create pathways in your home and avoiding having guests—you can obtain help from a psychologist or psychiatrist. It is not uncommon for compulsive hoarders to also experience tension in all manner of interpersonal relationships, low self-esteem, weak decision-making skills, poor social skills, and even occupational or legal issues. Treatment focuses on sorting items, developing decision-making skills, analyzing unwarranted emotional attachments, and curbing the acquisition of additional possessions.[7] If your symptoms are mild—in other words, if you're like most people—the ideas below will help clear your clutter and boost your energy immensely.

▲ ENERGY BOOSTER | Get rid of it

Unworn clothing, unwanted gifts, ancient paperwork—get rid of it. If you haven't used it in two years, ditch it, or pass it along in one of the following ways:

- Start a bag or box for charity; keep it in the basement or garage. There are so many worthy causes to choose from: Goodwill, women's organizations, Salvation Army, St. Vincent De Paul, church organizations. Add to your box or bag regularly. When it's full, take it with you to donate when you run errands. Get a receipt for your IRS records each time you drop off a donation.

- Sell it on eBay. If you don't have an eBay account, set one up on www.ebay.com. Locate all your possessions that have strong resale value but are of no use to you whatsoever and are only collecting dust. Take digital photographs of them. International commerce—what a fun way to get rid of duplicate or unwanted gifts. Turn your junk into money.

- Write a yard-sale date on the calendar. The kids can sell lemonade and get a nice little math lesson about making change, plus a little business lesson about earning a profit. Get the neighbors involved, and turn it into a fun multi-household yard sale to boost your profits even more. Donate whatever is left over to a local charity.

- At the office, keep only one hard copy of final documents. Recycle the rest. If you have a digital version, keep only the paper copy if required by company policy. Be sure to do a daily backup of all your computer files.

- Keep financial documents only as long as IRS regulations require. For tax returns, that's six years from the filing date. The same holds true for investment purchase and sale records, from the tax-filing deadline in the year of sale. Canceled checks and bank statements should likewise be kept for six years. Shred documents at home and at work that have become outdated. Devise a plan to repeat this process at the same time every year; just after New Year's Day is a great time, when you're in the mind-set of making a fresh start.

- For non-IRS documents at the office, decide how many years you'll keep things on file. Certain things may have historical value, such as annual reports. But for anything that doesn't possess inherent historical value, get rid of it. You don't need that coffee-stained piece of paper clip on it. Go through all your files and recycle everything that's now outside your time frame or from the woman who had your office before you. This will also prevent you from having to buy more and more filing cabinets, which also helps retain ample space. Again, devise a plan to repeat this process at the same time every year.

- Look at your possessions through your children's eyes. Pretend what it's going to be like for your children when you pass away and they have to sort through your belongings. Do you really need those love notes from sixth grade? The lock of your mother's baby hair? Keep it. Your grandmother's retro red diva suitcase? Keep it. Do you really need that box of photos from the junior high field trip? You're not even in any of the photos. Your children won't know who those people are.

▲ ▲ ▲
▼ ▼ ▼

▼ ENERGY BANDIT #6 | Not separating the treasures from the trash

Do you keep unwanted gifts due to a sense of guilt, simply because they're gifts? Do you have rented storage units to hold all the stuff you never use? Do you have boxes of things in your crawl space that you haven't used in years—if you even know what's in there? Worse yet, do you surround yourself with things that make you miserable? Do you keep a "thin section" in your closet? You know—the things you'll wear again once you lose twenty pounds? Every time you look at an item of clothing that doesn't fit, you feel deflated. Your energy plummets as you focus your attention on how fat you are versus finding something attractive that fits your "real" body.

▲ ENERGY BOOSTER | Accentuate the positive

There's a reason women burn photographs of their old boyfriends. If you're hoarding tangible proof of emotional baggage, you're sabotaging your energy, not to mention your mood. You're keeping that negativity hovering around your life. Clear the air. If there's one particle of anger attached to it, get rid of it. Why take up valuable space with outdated physical negativity? Don't keep mementos of failed relationships. If it's a legal issue such as a divorce or a custody dispute, keep only the bare minimum of final legal documents that you need. Out with the old, and in with the new.

▲ ▲ ▲
▼ ▼ ▼

▼ ENERGY BANDIT #7 | A disorganized office

No, a clean desk is not the sign of a simple mind. It's the sign of an efficient, energetic mind! The more space there is, the less crowded your energy is.

▲ ENERGY BOOSTER | Keep your office desk organized

Your desk should hold the computer monitor, keyboard, and mouse, plus any items that you use very frequently throughout the day, such as a stapler or calculator. If you absolutely must have a few pieces of paper for a particular project you're working on, create a file folder for each project. Label the tab with the project's name. Keep these in hanging files in a drawer in your desk. Each time you no longer need a piece of paper in a given folder, recycle it. And don't forget to keep your virtual desktop organized too. Follow these organizing guidelines:

- **File rather than pile.** If you have a cluttered office, you will spend more time trying to find information; you will have a harder time focusing on the task before you; other people won't be able to find anything; your system is in your head, which taxes your memory; you will have higher anxiety levels; and it could impede your career progression, as people perceive people with sloppy desks to have sloppy work. An organized desk sends this important message: I've got it together. Visualize your desk in your mind. What does it "say" to others? The next time someone walks over to your cluttered desk and makes a "joke" about the mess, you might want to listen and learn to file correctly. Your newly organized desk will now say that you are professional, competent, decisive, efficient, productive, and in control.
- **Don't use stackable trays.** Stackable trays are great near a printer to store frequently used letterheads, envelopes, and paper supplies. They are horrible, however, for active work, as they simply become storage areas for mystery piles. Once something goes into a stackable tray, it's typically "out of sight, out of mind." You'll end up with lower-priority items mixed in with high-priority work and project files mixed in with reference information. Instead, use vertical "step" files with colored file folders for each category of information you keep: projects, ideas, and subjects.
- **Put away future work.** Where do you put a meeting agenda for a meeting two weeks away? Where do you put an invoice so you remember to pay it in three weeks? Where do you put those plane tickets you don't want to lose? Where do you put the birthday card (that you managed to buy on time) so you remember to send it? If you're like most people, you put it on your desk. The piles of papers grow around you, as if you poured fertilizer on them. So what can you do instead? You need a system that will remind you which papers require your

action *today* and allow you to *forget* the rest until their time. The answer: a tickler file. Get forty-three hanging folders, label them 1–31 and January–December, and hang them in a drawer. File each piece of paper in the file of the day or month you need to see it again. Check your tickler file each day and pull out the items you filed. For example, if today were June 7, and you have a meeting on June 12, you would file the agenda in the folder marked "12."

- *Gather up your sticky notes.* Another area of organization has to do with all those little pink telephone slips, messages, and sticky notes you accumulate all day. Have you ever found yourself unable to understand your own scribbled notes or even to locate a message taken earlier in the day? Do you ever have trouble remembering if you returned a phone call or if someone called you back? Some people miss appointments or forget to return phone calls because they cannot locate the original message. Sticky notes are great to write down a fax number, mark a textbook, or jot a reminder to pick up dry cleaning. However, they should not be used for phone messages or anything requiring your action. Instead, use the "Tasks" or "To-do" function of your e-mail/calendaring software, or use an old-fashioned paper planner to write a list of things to do each day.

▲ ▲ ▲
▼ ▼ ▼

▼ ENERGY BANDIT #8 | Undone home-improvement projects

Nagging incomplete projects not only create clutter, but they also drag your mood down because another thing on your to-do list is staring you in the face.

▲ ENERGY BOOSTER | **Make a list of the projects you want to accomplish**

Finish that trim work on the hardwood floor you installed! Tend to that pile of mending! Mail that holiday cookie tin back to Aunt Bertha! If you actually wrote down an action for every item you usually just look at over and over, you could have fifty things to do. The trick is to pick one every day, week, or month, and systematically get them done. You'll see forward progress on your tasks by doing the following:

- Write a date on the calendar to finish any weekend projects. This is very helpful for home-improvement projects that you just can't get to on a weekday evening—items such as touching up paint, repairing tile grout, or installing a new section of baseboard. Then put away all those bags of home-improvement supplies that you've left out as a reminder; your date on the calendar will now be your reminder. You can get out the supplies when it's time to finish the project—and don't forget to put them away immediately afterward! Few to-do items hang over our heads and create more clutter than those regarding home improvement. This will clear the clutter, provide you with a big sense of relief and accomplishment, and boost your energy.
- Whenever possible, dispatch routine tasks immediately. If it takes less than three minutes, do it right then. Avoid saying "I'll do that later," as in "I'll take that off the wall later." Just walk down, get a screwdriver, and do it. Strive for NOW. Temporary places too often become permanent places. Put something away while it's in your hand rather than allowing large piles to accumulate.

▲ ▲ ▲

Conclusion

I was teaching a full-day seminar on time management. One of the participants complained several times that "This is so hard!" or "There's no way I could do that." After a while, it was quite apparent to me and his colleagues that while he wanted to change his behaviors, he had absolutely no faith in his ability to do so. I've never been one to tell people that being productive and energetic is easy. Sometimes it's downright hard. However, once you have systems in place and have enabled yourself to be productive, it's much easier in the long run.

But any type of change is hard. When learning new techniques, it's tempting to throw your hands up in despair and think, "There's no way I can do all this!" You can. You might just be stuck in a rut. You get into a certain routine and have fixed habits that are hard to break. You know you're not performing up to your ability, but hey, you're getting by, so it's good enough. You have to break out of your own self-limiting beliefs.

When you believe that something is impossible to do, you don't even try, or you do it halfheartedly, so that when it doesn't work, given your low level of effort, you say, "See, I told you I couldn't do it. It's impossible. I knew it was." This is the famous self-fulfilling prophecy. If you think you can get better and be more productive, you can, and you will.

Endnotes

One

1. American Psychological Association, "You're Getting Very Sleepy: More Sleep Would Make Most Americans Happier, Healthier and Safer," Psychology Matters, http://www.psychologymatters.org/sleep.html (retrieved January 13, 2007).

2. Kristyn Kusek Lewis, "Stay Healthy All Winter: Nine Proven Ways to Strengthen Your Immune System and Stop Getting Sick," Shape (December 2006): 88–91.

3. Michael Breus, "Sleep: More Important Than You Think," WebMD, 2004, http://www.webmd.com/content/article/64/72426.htm (retrieved January 13, 2007).

4. Lynn Lamberg, "Why Sleep Matters," National Sleep Foundation, http://www.sleepfoundation.org/hottopics/index.php?secid=15&id=293 (retrieved January 13, 2007).

5. American Academy of Sleep Medicine, "Sleep Hygiene: The Healthy Habits of Good Sleep," SleepEducation, 2005, http://www.sleepeducation.com/Hygiene.aspx (retrieved February 24, 2007).

6. "Sleep Disorders and Problems: Symptoms, Tests, and Treatment," Helpguide, http://www.helpguide.org/life/sleep_disorders.htm (retrieved January 13, 2007).

7. "Sleep Disorders—Types and Symptoms," Neurology Channel, http://www.neurologychannel.com/sleepdisorders/types.shtml (retrieved January 13, 2007).

8. National Sleep Disorders Research Plan, "Normal Sleep, Sleep Restriction and Health Consequences," National Heart Blood and Lung Institute, http://www.nhlbi.nih.gov/health/prof/sleep/res_plan/section4/section4.html (retrieved January 13, 2007).

9. Michael Breus, "Sleep: More Important Than You Think," WebMD,

2004, http://www.webmd.com/content/article/64/72426.htm (retrieved January 13, 2007).

10. Monash University Centre of Obesity Research and Education, "Losing Weight for a Better Night's Sleep," *International Journal of Obesity* (May 26, 2005). From http://www.monash.edu.au/ (retrieved January 13, 2007).

11. Norman Wilder, "Obstructive Sleep Apnea," SleepEducation.com, January 12, 2006, http://sleepeducation.com/Disorder.aspx?id=7 (retrieved January 13, 2007).

12. Columbia University, "Sleep More to Gain Less," America Online, http://www.aol.com (retrieved January 20, 2005).

13. American Academy of Family Physicians, "Seasonal Affective Disorder," FamilyDoctor, September 2005, http://familydoctor.org/267.xml (retrieved February 5, 2007).

Two

1. Department of Health and Human Services (HHS) and Department of Agriculture (USDA), "Dietary Guidelines for Americans 2005," chapter 4, Healthier U.S. gov, January 12, 2005, http://www.healthierus.gov/dietaryguidelines/ (retrieved January 13, 2007).

2. Cynthia Sass, "7 Diet Rules You Must Break: Following These Everyday Conventions Will Make You Fat. Ditch 'em and Lose Weight!" *Shape* (September 2005), 92.

3. United States Department of Agriculture, "Inside the Pyramid," MyPyramid.gov, January 12, 2005, http://www.mypyramid.gov/pyramid/index.html (retrieved January 3, 2007).

4. Nicole Diliberti, Peter L. Bordi, Martha T. Conklin, Liane S. Roe, and Barbara J. Rolls, "Increased Portion Size Leads to Increased Energy Intake in a Restaurant Meal," The Obesity Society, January 15, 2004, http://www.obesityresearch.org/cgi/content/full/12/3/562 (retrieved January 13, 2007).

5. S. Liao, "Your Holiday Survival Guide," *Shape* (December 2006): 92.

6. Rob Medich, "Choose Your Takeout Wisely," AOL Diet and Fitness, http://diets.aol.com/newsandtrends/ (retrieved January 13, 2007).

Three

1. Recommended Daily Allowance, in milligrams (mg) or micrograms (μg).
2. Ben Best, "Fats You Need—Essential Fatty Acids," Ben Best Health, http://www.benbest.com/health/essfat.html (retrieved January 17, 2007).
3. Vitamins and Health Supplements Guide, http://www.vitamins-supplements.org (retrieved January 17, 2007).
4. Mary Kay Mitchell, *Nutrition Across the Life Span* (Philadelphia, PA: W.B. Saunders, 1997). From Questia, http://www.questia.com/PM.qst?a=o&d=104079454 (retrieved January 19, 2007).
5. Especially critical for the health of women.
6. National Library of Medicine, "Dehydration," MedlinePlus, June 13, 2006, http://www.nlm.nih.gov/medlineplus/ency/article/000982.htm#visualContent (retrieved January 18, 2007).
7. Andrew P. Jenkins, "Herbal Energizers: Speed by Any Other Name," *JOPERD—The Journal of Physical Education, Recreation & Dance* 68.2 (1997): 39+. From Questia, http://www.questia.com/PM.qst?a=o&d=5002229997 (retrieved January 19, 2007).
8. Ibid.
9. Mim J. Landry, *Understanding Drugs of Abuse: The Processes of Addiction, Treatment, and Recovery* (Washington, DC: American Psychiatric Press, 1994), 8.

Four

1. "Physical Activity for Everyone: The Importance of Physical Activity," Centers for Disease Control, http://www.cdc.gov/nccdphp/dnpa/physical/importance/index.htm (retrieved January 17, 2007).
2. C. M. Bernaards, et al., "Can Strenuous Leisure Time Physical Activity Prevent Psychological Complaints in a Working Population?" Occupa-

tional and Environmental Medicine, 2006. http://oem.bmj.com/cgi/content/full/63/1/10.

3. "Aerobic Exercise: What 30 Minutes a Day Can Do for Your Body," Mayo Clinic, http://www.mayoclinic.com/health/aerobic-exercise/EP00002 (retrieved January 13, 2007).

4. Sharon Begley, "How to Keep Your Aging Brain Fit: Aerobics," *The Wall Street Journal*, November 16, 2006, D1.

5. Tara Parker-Pope, "Why Your New Year's Resolution to Get Healthier May Be Pretty Easy to Keep," *The Wall Street Journal*, January 2006. From http://www.ltwell.com/wall_street_journal.htm (retrieved January 13, 2007).

6. Renee Cloe, "Dieting and Metabolism," Primusweb, http://www.primusweb.com/fitnesspartner/library/weight/0698metabolism.htm (retrieved February 7, 2007).

7. Suzanne Schlosberg, *Fitness for Travelers: The Ultimate Workout Guide for the Road* (Boston: Houghton Mifflin Company, 2002), 30.

Five

1. Dr. Chris Melby, "Does Exercise Affect Resting Metabolism?" About Sports Medicine, http://sportsmedicine.about.com/od/anatomyandphysiology/a/rmr.htm (retrieved February 7, 2007).

2. Richard K. Bernstein, *Dr. Bernstein's Diabetes Solution* (New York: Little, Brown, 2005), 41.

3. Dixie Farley, "Top 10 Laboratory Tests: Blood Will Tell," *FDA Consumer* (July–August 1989): 22+. From Questia, http://www.questia.com/PM.qst?a=o&d=5002147508 (retrieved January 27, 2007).

4. Cynthia Sass, "7 Diet Rules You Must Break: Following These Everyday Conventions Will Make You Fat. Ditch 'em and Lose Weight!" *Shape* (September 2005), 198.

5. Christine Gorman, "Why We Sleep," *Time*, December 20, 2004, 52.

6. Ibid.

7. Colette Bouchez, "Top 10 Ways to Boost Your Energy," WebMD, Au-

gust 19, 2005, http://www.webmd.com/content/article/110/109604.htm
(retrieved February 5, 2007).

Six

1. Susie Stephenson, "When Computers Attack: Electromagnetic Radiation," School of Library, Archival, and Information Studies, December 6, 2002, http://www.slais.ubc.ca/courses/libr500/02-03-wt1/www/A_Davis/radiation.htm (retrieved February 23, 2007).
2. Peter McLaughlin, *CatchFire: A 7-Step Program to Ignite Energy, Defuse Stress, and Power Boost Your Career* (New York: Random House, 1997), 133.
3. Ibid.
4. Dr. Chris Melby, "Does Exercise Affect Resting Metabolism?" September 2004, About Sports Medicine http://sportsmedicine.about.com/od/anatomyandphysiology/a/rmr.htm (retrieved February 7, 2007).
5. E.g., Abitbol M. Maurice, "Effect of Posture and Locomotion on Energy Expenditure," *American Journal of Physical Anthropology* 77.2 (1988): 191–99.
6. Jim Loehr and Tony Schwartz, *The Power of Full Engagement* (New York: Free Press, 2003).
7. Not to be confused with "biorhythms," which is a term used to designate the unsubstantiated theory that cyclic variations in behavior are related to a person's birth date and astrological sign.
8. "Lithium Blocks Enzyme to Help Cells' Clocks Keep on Tickin'," National Institute of Mental Health, http://www.nimh.nih.gov/press/lithiumenzyme.cfm (retrieved February 11, 2007).

Seven

1. "Oral Health Information for the Public," American Academy of Periodontology, Frequently Asked Questions, September 13, 2006, http://www.perio.org/consumer/media/media-faq.htm (retrieved January 13, 2007).

2. Karen Pallarito, "Health Maladies Cost Billions in Lost Productivity," Prevent Disease, http://preventdisease.com/news/articles/maladies_productivity.shtml (retrieved January 13, 2007).

3. Arizona Venture Capital, Matrixx Initiatives, Inc., Updates Sales and Earnings Guidance, January 5, 2007, http://azventurecapital.com/arizona-venture-capital/venture-capital-news/matrixx-initiatives-inc-updates-sales-and-earnings-guidance/ (retrieved January 13, 2007).

4. Betty McElroy and Shelley Miller, "Effectiveness of Zinc Gluconate Glycine Lozenges (Cold-Eeze) Against the Common Cold in School-Aged Subjects," *American Journal of Therapeutics* 9(6) (2002):472–75. From http://www.americantherapeutics.com (retrieved January 13, 2007).

5. "First In-Office Study Dishes the Dirt on Desks," *Marketwire News,* April 15, 2002, http://www.marketwire.com/mw/release_html_bl?release_id=40596 (retrieved January 13, 2007).

6. "10 Other Paths to Better Health," *Health and Behavior, USA Today,* July 12, 2005. From http://www.usatoday.com/news/health/2005-07-12-10-other-paths_x.htm (retrieved January 13, 2007).

7. Kataria Madhuri, "Benefits of Laughter Yoga," Laughter Yoga, http://www.laughteryoga.org/about-benefits-laughter.php (retrieved February 6, 2007).

8. "An Introduction to Indoor Air Quality," U.S. Environmental Protection Agency, http://www.epa.gov/iaq/voc.html (retrieved January 13, 2007).

Eight

1. National Center for Health Statistics, NCHS Health E Stats, January 11, 2007, http://www.cdc.gov/nchs/products/pubs/pubd/hestats/3and4/sedentary.htm (retrieved February 5, 2007).

2. V. Lohr, "Indoor Plants Increase Worker Productivity," Dr. Delphinium, 2007, http://www.drdelphinium.com/green/research.asp (retrieved February 6, 2007).

3. Katy Chamberlin, "8 Laws of Natural Health—Air," Amazing Health, http://www.amazinghealth.org/articles-general%20principles-8laws-air.htm (retrieved February 7, 2007).

4. "Environmental Psychologists Investigate Motivations and Strategies that Help People Sustain Regular Walking Routines," University of Michigan School of Natural Resources and Environment, November 20, 2006, http://www.snre.umich.edu/news/details.php?id=1523 (retrieved February 5, 2007).

5. Thomas Nielsen and Karsten Hansen, "Nearby Nature and Green Areas Encourage Outdoor Activities and Decrease Mental Stress," CAB Reviews: Perspectives Agriculture, Veterinary Science, Nutrition and Natural Resources, http://www.cababstractsplus.org/cabreviews/Reviews.asp?action= display&openMenu=relatedItems&ReviewID= 25640&Year=2006 (retrieved February 7, 2007).

6. Katy Chamberlin, "Eight Laws of Health," Amazing Health, http://www.amazinghealth.org/articles-general%20principles-8laws-sun.htm (retrieved February 16, 2007).

7. A.D.A.M., Inc., "Yoga," University of Maryland Medical Center, 2004, http://www.umm.edu/altmed/ConsModalities/Yogacm.html (retrieved February 6, 2007).

8. "TCM This Season," Traditional Chinese Medicine World Foundation, 2006, http://tcmworld.org/publications/harmony/winter_2006/h4-winter/ (retrieved February 6, 2007).

9. Michael Gach, *Acupressure's Potent Points: A Guide to Self-Care for Common Ailments* (New York: Bantam Books, 1990), 20.

10. ICBS, Inc., "Meditation Techniques: Transcendental Meditation," 1st Holistic, 2007, http://1stholistic.com/Meditation/hol_meditation_TM.htm (retrieved February 5, 2007).

11. "Foot Problems in Women: High Heels and Your Health," Mayo Clinic, April 21, 2006, http://www.mayoclinic.com/health/foot-problems/WO00114 (retrieved February 6, 2007).

12. Enzo Sella, "High Heels Dangerous to Your Health," Yale–New Haven Hospital, June 4, 2001, http://www.ynhh.org/healthlink/womens/womens_6_01.html (retrieved February 6, 2007).

13. "The Bra and Health Risks," Earth Wisdom, 2005 http://www.menstrual-cycle-period.com/bra_health.htm (retrieved February 6, 2007).

Nine

1. Thich Nhat Hanh, *Anger* (New York: Riverhead Books, 2001), 178.
2. Bryan Robinson, Jane Carroll, and Claudia Flowers, "Marital Estrangement, Positive Affect, and Locus of Control Among Spouses of Workaholics and Spouses of Non-workaholics: A National Study," *American Journal of Family Therapy* 29 (October 1, 2001): 397–410.

Ten

1. Claudia Wallis, "The New Science of Happiness," *Time*, January 17, 2005. From http://www.reflectivehappiness.com/AboutUs/TimeMagazine/ (retrieved January 13, 2007).

Eleven

1. Eli Finkel, Amy Dalton, Amy Brunell, Sarah Scarbeck, and Tanya Chartrand, "High-Maintenance Interaction: Inefficient Social Coordination Impairs Self-Regulation," *Journal of Personality and Social Psychology* 91, No. 3 (2006): 456–75.

Fourteen

1. John J. Ratey, *A User's Guide to the Brain: Perception, Attention, and the Four Theaters of the Brain* (New York: Vintage, 2002). From eNotAlone, http://www.enotalone.com/article/6232.html (retrieved February 2, 2007).
2. "Salary Is Rarely the Reason for Leaving a Job, Executives Say," HRMarketer, http://www.hrmarketer.com/home/newsviewer.php?ppa= 6prjo%60%5BghlnjgmWUie%7D38%7Dbfem%5E (retrieved February 2, 2007).
3. Aviva Patz, "A Simple 4-Week Plan to Make Over Your Health," *Shape* (October 2006): 112.
4. Mihaly Csikszentmihalyi, *Flow: The Psychology of Optimal Experience* (New York: Harper and Row, 1990), 29.
5. "7 Benefits of Reading Fiction," Buzzle: Intelligent Life on the Web,

http://www.buzzle.com/editorials/8-22-2005-75260.asp (retrieved February 5, 2007).

6. Russell A. Ward, Mark La Gory, and Susan R. Sherman, *The Environment for Aging: Interpersonal, Social, and Spatial Contexts* (Tuscaloosa, AL: University of Alabama, 1988), 108–12.

Fifteen

1. Laura Baron, "The Economics of Ergonomics," *Journal of Accountancy* 202.6 (2006): 34–39.

2. Paul McFedries, "BlackBerry Thumb," *Word Spy*, 2006, http://www.wordspy.com/words/blackberrythumb.asp (retrieved January 13, 2007).

3. Sally O'Reilly, "Let There Be Light," *Personnel Today* (October 31, 2006): 28.

4. There is a real Sumatran product called Kopi Luwak that costs about three hundred dollars per pound. No, really!

5. "Norwalk City Employee Sues over Smells," Free Republic, March 1, 2005, http://www.freerepublic.com/focus/f-news/1353308/posts (retrieved January 17, 2007).

6. Teresa Witham, "HR in Brief: Turn Up the Thermostat," *Credit Union Management* (February 2007): 40.

7. "Color Me Productive: Research Gauges Impact of Color in the Workplace," University of Texas at Austin, http://www.utexas.edu/supportut/news_pub/yg_kwallek-color.html (retrieved March 1, 2007).

8. "Electromagnetic Radiation and Computers," UCLA Ergonomics http://ergonomics.ucla.edu/articles/EMRandComp.pdf (retrieved March 1, 2007).

9. "Eyestrain and Your Computer Screen: Tips for Getting Relief," Mayo Clinic, http://www.mayoclinic.com/health/eyestrain/WL00060 (retrieved March 1, 2007).

10. "The Impact of Ventilation Control Methods on Worker Productivity," UC Berkeley Building Science, http://arch.ced.berkeley.edu/resources/bldgsci/research/impact.htm (retrieved March 1, 2007).

11. William J. Fisk, "Health and Productivity Gains from Better Indoor

Environments and Their Implications for the U.S. Department of Energy,"
Rand Corporation, http://www.rand.org/scitech/stpi/Evision/
Supplement/fisk.pdf (retrieved March 1, 2007).

12. "Stress on the Brain," The Franklin Institute Resources for Science
Learning, 2004, http://www.fi.edu/brain/stress.htm (retrieved February 5,
2007).

13. "Minimizing Noise Stress," Stress Management Tips and Techniques,
MindTools, http://www.mindtools.com/stress/EnvironmentalStress/
NoiseStress.htm (retrieved February 5, 2007).

14. "Stress on the Brain."

15. Ibid.

Sixteen

1. Anna Hansson, Pernilla Hilleras, and Yvonne Forsell, "What Kind of
Self-Care Strategies Do People Report Using and Is There an Association
with Well-being?" *Social Indicators Research* 73 (2005): 133–39.

2. "Friendship: Your Key to a Healthy Lifestyle," Health Expressions,
2007, http://www.healthexpressions.com/family_friends/index_sep2005
.shtml (retrieved February 19, 2007).

3. "Social Phobia (Social Anxiety Disorder)," Brain Physics Mental
Health Resource, 2007, http://www.brainphysics.com/social-phobia.php
(retrieved February 20, 2007).

4. "Friends Help People Live Longer," BBC News, June 15, 2005, http://
news.bbc.co.uk/2/hi/health/4094632.stm (retrieved February 19, 2007).

5. Rebecca Sweat, "Frenzied Families," Vision Media, 2002, http://
vision.org/visionmedia/article.aspx?id=244 (retrieved February 5, 2007).

6. Ibid.

Seventeen

1. Hughes M. Helm, Judith C. Hays, Elizabeth P. Flint, Harold G. Koenig,
and Dan G. Blazer, "Does Private Religious Activity Prolong Survival?"
The Journals of Gerontology Series A: Biological Sciences and Medical Sci-

ences 55 (2000). From http://biomed.gerontologyjournals.org (retrieved January 13, 2007).

2. Research at TRI, Touch Research Institute, http://www6.miami.edu/touch-research/research.htm (retrieved January 13, 2007).

3. Kristyn Kusek Lewis, "Stay Healthy All Winter: Nine Proven Ways to Strengthen Your Immune System and Stop Getting Sick," *Shape* (December 2006): 88–91.

4. "Bioenergetics," American Cancer Society, http://www.cancer.org/docroot/ETO/content/ETO_5_3X_Bioenergetics.asp?sitearea=ETO (retrieved February 24, 2007).

5. Beverly Beuermann-King, "Handling Job Stress," Work Smart, Live Smart, http://www.worksmartlivesmart.com/files/documents/public/Handling%20Job%20Stress.pdf (retrieved February 24, 2007).

6. Ian Towers, Linda Duxbury, Christopher Higgins, and John Thomas, "Time Thieves and Space Invaders: Technology, Work, and the Organization," *Journal of Organizational Change Management* 19.5 (2006): 593–618.

7. "Adrenaline Junkie," Wikipedia, http://en.wikipedia.org/wiki/Adrenaline_junkie (retrieved February 24, 2007).

8. Meyer Friedman and Ray H. Rosenman, *Type A Behavior and Your Heart* (New York: Fawcett Crest Books, 1974).

Eighteen

1. "Nielsen Reports Americans Watch TV at Record Levels," Nielsen Media Research News Release, September 29, 2005, www.nielsenmedia.com.

2. Joseph Mercola, "TV Watching, Childhood Obesity Linked," The Best Natural Health Information and Newsletter, http://www.mercola.com/1998/archive/tv_and_obesity_in_children.htm (retrieved February 5, 2007).

3. Robert Roy Britt, "Drivers on Cell Phones Kill Thousands, Snarl Traffic," Live Science, February 1, 2005, http://www.livescience.com/technology/050201_cell_danger.html (retrieved February 16, 2007).

4. Cheri Speier, Joseph Valacich, and Iris Vessey, "The Effects of Task In-

terruption and Information Presentation on Individual Decision Making," Interruptions, http://interruptions.net/literature/Speier-ICIS97-p21-speier.pdf (retrieved February 5, 2007).

Nineteen

1. Kristin Perrone, Kay Webb, Stephen Wright, Vance Jackson, and Tracy Ksiazak, "Relationship of Spirituality to Work and Family Roles and Life Satisfaction," *Journal of Mental Health Counseling* 28 (2006): 253–68.

Twenty-one

1. "Feng shui," Wikipedia, http://en.wikipedia.org/wiki/Feng_shui (retrieved February 13, 2007).
2. Rodika Tchi, "Clear the Clutter with Feng Shui," About, http://fengshui.about.com/od/thebasics/qt/clearclutter.htm (retrieved February 13, 2007).
3. Ibid.
4. Ibid.
5. Ibid.
6. M. Williams, "What Is Compulsive Hoarding?" BrainPhysics, 2000, http://www.brainphysics.com/hoarding.php (retrieved February 13, 2007).
7. "Compulsive Hoarding," Bio-Behavioral Institute, http://www.bio-behavioral.com/hoarding.asp (retrieved February 13, 2007).

Laura Stack, MBA, CSP, is a professional speaker and personal productivity expert who helps people leave the office earlier, with less stress, and greater results to show for it. Laura is the president of The Productivity Pro®, Inc., which is a Denver-based training firm specializing in productivity improvement in high-stress organizations. She is one of a handful of professional speakers whose business focuses solely on time management and productivity topics. Since 1992, Laura has taught her original principles on improving output, lowering stress, and saving time in today's workplaces.

Laura holds an MBA in organizational management (University of Colorado, 1991), integrating the importance of productivity in business with employee retention and satisfaction. She is also on the board of directors of the National Speakers Association (NSA) and is the recipient of the Certified Speaking Professional (CSP) award, NSA's highest earned designation, held by less than 10 percent of professional speakers worldwide. Laura is a certified specialist in Microsoft Office Outlook and was awarded a Board Approval in Productivity Improvement from the Society for the Advancement of Consulting (SAC).

Laura is the best-selling author or coauthor of five books, including *Find More Time* (Broadway Books, 2006); *Leave the Office Earlier* (Broadway Books, 2004), which was hailed as "the best of the bunch" by the *New York Times* and listed on the June 2004 Book Sense Business and Economics Bestseller list; and two of the popular *Chicken Soup for the Soul* books. *Leave the Office Earlier* has been published in seven countries and in five foreign languages—Japanese, Korean, Chinese, Taiwanese, and Italian. Laura's popular monthly electronic newsletter has subscribers in thirty-eight countries.

Widely regarded as one of the leading experts in the field of employee productivity and workplace issues, she has been featured nationally on the CBS *Early Show*, CNN, NPR, Bloomberg radio, NBC TV news, WB news, the *New York Times*, *USA Today*, Washington Post.com, the *Chicago Tribune*, *SELF*, *ME*, *Working Mother*, *Bottom Line Personal*, *Ladies' Home Journal*, *Redbook*, *Entrepreneur*, *Reader's Digest*, *Cosmopolitan*, *Woman's Day*, and *Parents*.

Laura draws from her background as a corporate manager, a University of Colorado instructor, a CareerTrack speaker, a radio talk-show host, a newspaper columnist, and a small-business owner. Her client list reads like a *Who's Who* of recognizable Fortune 500 companies, including Microsoft, IBM, GM, KPMG, Cisco, Coors, the Denver Broncos, Lockheed Martin, Lucent Technologies, Wells Fargo, Mobil, Time Warner, and Visa, plus a multitude of associations and governmental agencies.

Laura lives with her husband and three children in Denver, Colorado.

Contact information:

Laura Stack, MBA, CSP
The Productivity Pro®, Inc.
9948 S. Cottoncreek Drive
Highlands Ranch, CO 80130
Phone: 303–471–7401
Fax: 303–471–7402
www.TheProductivityPro.com
Laura@TheProductivityPro.com

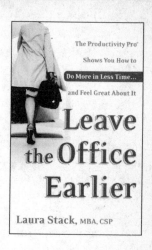
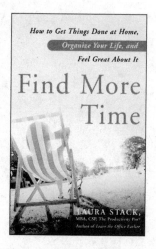